Selected Topics in Exercise Cardiology and Rehabilitation

ETTORE MAJORANA INTERNATIONAL SCIENCE SERIES
Series Editor:
Antonino Zichichi
European Physical Society
Geneva, Switzerland

(LIFE SCIENCES)

Volume 1   BLADDER TUMORS AND OTHER TOPICS IN UROLOGICAL
ONCOLOGY
Edited by M. Pavone-Macaluso, P. H. Smith, and F. Edsmyr

Volume 2   ADVANCES IN RADIATION PROTECTION AND DOSIMETRY
IN MEDICINE
Edited by Ralph H. Thomas and Victor Perez-Mendez

Volume 3   PULMONARY CIRCULATION IN HEALTH AND DISEASE
Edited by G. Cumming and G. Bonsignore

Volume 4   SELECTED TOPICS IN EXERCISE CARDIOLOGY
AND REHABILITATION
Edited by A. Raineri, J. J. Kellermann, and V. Rulli

Volume 5   THE AGING BRAIN: Neurological and Mental Disturbances
Edited by G. Barbagallo-Sangiorgi and A. N. Exton-Smith

Selected Topics in Exercise Cardiology and Rehabilitation

Edited by
A. Raineri

Cattedra di Fisiopatologia Cardiovascolare
Università di Palermo, Policlinico
Palermo, Italy

J. J. Kellermann

Cardiac Evaluation and Rehabilitation Institute
The Chaim Sheba Medical Center
Tel Hashomer, Israel

and
V. Rulli

Centro Malattie Cardiovascolari
Ospedale S. Camillo
Rome, Italy

Springer Science+Business Media, LLC

Library of Congress Cataloging in Publication Data

Course on Functional Evaluation and Rehabilitation in Cardiology, 1st, Erice, Italy,
  1979.
  Selected topics in exercise cardiology and rehabilitation.

  (Ettore Majorana international science series: Life sciences; v. 4)
  Sponsored by the International School of Cardiology at Ettore Majorana.
  Includes index.
    1. Heart—Diseases—Diagnosis—Congresses. 2. Exercise tests—Congresses. 3. Car-
  diacs—Rehabilitation—Congresses. I. Raineri, A. II. Kellermann, Jan J. III. Rulli,
  V. IV. International School of Cardiology. [DNLM: 1. Coronary disease—Rehabilita-
  tion—Congresses. 2. Heart diseases—Rehabilitation—Congresses. 3. Exercise test—
  Congresses. 4. Exercise therapy—Congresses. W1 ET712M v. 4/ WG200 C861 1979s]
  RC683.5.E94C68 1979   616.1'2'0624   80-19841
  ISBN 978-1-4684-3856-7   ISBN 978-1-4684-3854-3 (eBook)
  DOI 10.1007/978-1-4684-3854-3

Proceedings of the First Course on Functional Evaluation and
Rehabilitation in Cardiology, held in
Erice, Sicily, Italy, October 15-20, 1979.

©1980 Springer Science+Business Media New York
Originally published by Plenum Press, New York in 1980
Softcover reprint of the hardcover 1st edition 1980

PREFACE

In this book the lectures of the first course of the International School of Cardiology at Ettore Majorana are presented.

It is difficult to reflect in a publication of this kind the atmosphere and spirit of this postgraduate course. Moreover, the beautiful scenery of Erice and its surroundings, celebrated by ancient Greek poets, can never be described by the editors of this book.

The purpose of this course was to deepen our knowledge accumulated todate on the subjects of non-invasive cardio-circulatory assessment and the analysis of the comprehensive approach to cardiac rehabilitation. The clinical value of exercise testing, echo-cardiography, scintigraphy, systolic time intervals have been discussed, as well as the tasks of exercise training, surgery and drugs in the secondary prevention of coronary heart disease. The problems of arrhythmias and the prevention of sudden death have been touched on, as well as early mobilization after myocardial infarction, the use of digoxin and beta blockers and finally, the controversies in cardiac rehabilitation.

It was a great challenge and pleasure for the program directors of this course to act as moderators. After a careful analysis of the performance of the faculty and the response of the participants, we came to the conclusion that the success of this course went beyond our expectations. The close constructive cooperation between faculty and participants was one of the clues of the course. The scientific standards maintained were the result of interactions between the quality of the lectures and the high professional level of the participants.

Perhaps the most important part of this course was the frank and critical exchange of views during discussions. A number of changes and possible improvements have been suggested by the

participants and these will be taken into consideration in the
next course, such as an early presentation of abstracts.

Finally, we sould like to express our gratitude to the
sponsoring bodies, the directors of the Center, Professor
Zichichi and the secretary of Ettore Majorana, Dr. Gabriele.

The director of the School, Professor Raineri and his staff,
worked in very close cooperation with the program directors and
without their intensive assistance and guidance the course could
not have been organized.

We hope that the next course will meet the expectations of
the participants and reach the targets of the faculty.

Jan J. Kellermann
Vincenzo Rulli

Directors of the Course on
Functional Evaluation and
Rehabilitation in Cardiology

INTRODUCTION

Since 1963 the "Ettore Majorana Centre" has received at Erice outstanding scientists from all over the world, and it can be proud for holding a meeting of such a high level.

I would like to thank in particular the directors of the course, Prof. Kellermann and Prof. Rulli, who have played an essential part in the scientific organization of the 1st Course on Functional Evaluation and Rehabilitation in Cardiology. The international prestige they have in our field could have been a valid premise, but without their efforts it would have been impossible to obtain these results.

I would also like to thank all lecturers, who by accepting our invitation, have shown a great sensitivity.

Prof. A. Zichichi, founder and director of this Centre, president of the European Society of Physics, director of the Nuclear Research Centre in Geneva, and a world known scientist, who for years has been carrying out qualified work in favour of culture, says: man needs a cultural revival. Logic was discovered 3,000 years ago; science, which is the logic of nature, 350 years ago; but the so called modern man still remains at the cultural level of speech. Moreover, if science continued to produce more science without making culture, the actual gap would become an unfilled depth and the ivory towers less and less towers and more and more ghettos.

The School of Cardiology moves in the direction of this modern culture.

The technological progress has allowed notable developments of knowledge, but we must also admit that often it is labelled as progress what can be only called novelty.

In this logic, to do what others haven't yet done can give way to disastrous results.

Only the support of a really modern culture, can be capable of influencing the methods and prospects of science made to measure to man, who is made a slave by technological progress and by the novelties.

It is just in this light that this 1st Course begins, finding in the topics for discussion a sure occasion for showing it.

The rehabilitation of the heart patient can't avoid a valid basis of knowledge, which is culture, if one wants to be certain to influence in a sensible manner the complete balance, not only physical, of the patient, who, because he is a human being, needs to feel valid and useful, in the perspective of his own active social participation. But the task of this Course can't end in a simple, even if highly meritorious, transfer of knowledge. The experiences made by each of us in his own Institution can become the more useful the more one is capable of giving others the possibility to know the means and the procedures through which a result can be obtained. In such a philosophy, this Erice meeting may become a School.

I would like to wish everybody useful work in this peaceful Centre, suitable for meditation.

Angelo Raineri
Director of International
School of Cardiology
"Ettore Majorana" Centre

CONTENTS

CARDIAC REHABILITATION : AN OVERVIEW

H. Denolin

Hôpital Universitaire Saint-Pierre
Brussels

PLACE AND DEFINITION OF CARDIAC REHABILITATION

We know, from the data published by WHO, that cardiovascular diseases can be considered to be the major cause of death. In 1967, for about 50 countries, cardiovascular diseases were responsible for 37% of all deaths; ischemic heart disease (I.H.D.) accounted for about 75% of these deaths, and this is not related to the ageing of the population (1). In spite of a regression in the number of deaths by IHD in USA during the last years (2), and probably in some countries of Europe, the cardio-vascular diseases remain the first cause of death in many countries. This means that all the aspects of the fight against these diseases should be considered : primary prevention, medical and surgical treatment, but also the reduction of the impact of IHD on the patient and on the community. This last approach is the task of Rehabilitation.

A definition of cardiac rehabilitation was proposed by a working group of WHO : "The rehabilitation of cardiac patients can be defined as the sum of activities required to ensure them the best possible physical, mental and social conditions so that they may, by their own efforts, resume as normal a place as possible in the life of the community (3)." The report continues: "Rehabilitation should take place at an early stage and be continuous. The doctor must bear it in mind from his very first contact with the patient and not lose sight of it in any of the phases of treatment or supervision. Every aspect of the patient must be taken into account in rehabilitaiton, including his physiological, clinical , psychological and social problems. Lastly, rehabilitation cannot be regarded as an isolated form of

1

therapy, but must be integrated with the whole treatment of which it constitutes only one facet" (3). These definitions proposed in 1967, remain completely valid to day.

Up to now, rehabilitation was considered principally in coronary diseases, and chiefly after myocardial infarction, and the following pages deal with this disease; but most of the cardio-vascular diseases need the same approach.

At the beginning of the rehabilitation era, the interest was focused on the physical condition of the patient; later, the psychological problem were included in the programme, and more recently the secondary prevention was introduced as an important part of the fight against the disease. Today, a complete and comprehensive approach of the patient is considered as a necessity. But, for practical reasons, the different parts of a rehabilitation programme will be separated in this paper.

It is also useful, for the same practical reasons, to divide the evolution of a myocardial infarction in different phases: i) from the acute attack to the end of hospitalization; ii) convalescence period of 4 to 12 weeks; iii) return to a normal life or, if needed, improvement of the physical and psychological situation; iv) consolidation, permanent treatment or supervision.

PHYSICAL ACTIVITY AFTER MYOCARDIAL INFARCTION

When, in 1802, W. Heberden described angina pectoris, he also noticed that the condition of one of his patients suffering from angina was much improved by sawing wood for half an hour every day. This very first observation was neglected and when, in the first half of the present century, myocardial infarction was defined, the opinion of a need for a prolonged bed rest and a definitive incapacity was accepted.

Mobilization during the First Weeks

For pathologists, absolute and prolonged rest was regarded as a requirement for the healing of the lesions, and for the development of collateral circulation, and reintegration into active life was considered as undesirable.

In 1944, Levine reported the harmful effects of supine rest in some cardiac diseases and stressed the fact that the upright position diminished the venous return, and hence decreased the cardiac workload, and that at the same time the patient's psychological condition was improved.

In 1952, Levine and Lown have shown that during the first week following a myocardial infarction, the rest in the armchair was beneficial and without risk (4). But a mobilization before

the first six weeks, as traditional, has only been accepted very
gradually.

Today, an "early" mobilization is recommended and the
unfavourable effects of a prolonged immobilization are well
known (5). But, when looking through the literature, it appears
that the meaning of the work "early" may be quite different from
one center to another. If it is generally accepted that a
mobilization in bed should start after one or two days in non
complicated cases, the duration of hospitalization remains
strongly different.

The present attitude, an "early" mobilization or "early"
discharge from the hospital, remains based on empirical
observations by the clinicians, and no systematic study was made
for definition of the optimal duration of bed rest or hospitalization;
this is probably partly related to the lack of good short term
prognostic indexes: we have no clear-cut criteria to decide upon
the optimal moment of discharge of an individual patient. But,
apparently, in cases with good clinical evolution, a discharge
after 8 to 10 days does not seem harmful. An early evaluation of
the physical condition by an exercise test, after 7 to 10 days,
could be of interest; this is apparently a logical approach as it
makes possible an objective evaluation of the patient's
cardiovascular response to a graded exercise and permit to unmask
signs of intolerance to activity, especially dysrhythmia.
Preliminary studies, with a follow up of 2 months, with a control
group, demonstrate that this early testing is without any risk
when the contraindications and the criteria for stopping are
respected (6). But there is an urgent need for further studies,
with a long term follow up, to establish all the methodological
aspects of early exercise tests, their contra-indications and
their prognostic value.

So we can conclude that physical rehabilitation during the
first days or weeks after a myocardial infarction remains still
at an experimental stage as far as all the details are concerned.

Reduced hospitalization, early mobilization and early testing
are trends, and should not yet be changed in strict rules before
a good evaluation of the results of different programmes: it
is important to go on with the current clinical studies, with
criticism, in order to avoid the introduction of a renewed
empirism or dogmatic statement. The problems open for research
are: the exact evaluation of the severity of the disease, the
optimal moment for mobilization, the physical training during the
first weeks, the optimal duration of hospitalization, and the right
time for first evaluation of the residual physical capacity.

Training during Convalescence

     More intensive training after a few weeks following myocardial
infarction has now become a common practice, sometimes even
considered as a new religion. The physiological effects of this
kind of training remain debated, but are positive in terms of an
increased performance and an increased maximal oxygen consumption.
But the optimal duration of the programme of training, the intensity
of exercise and the number of sessions remain oper for discussion.

     Little is known up to now on the influence of physical training
on morbidity: some authors have reported no effects on both,
although others have shown a decreased mortality rate. But
whatever the beneficial effect of physical exercise on the patient's
condition might be, it is generally accepted that the psychological
influence of physical activity is of great importance (7).

     Despite the generalization of the training programme, the
selection of patients require additional information, to ensure the
patient's compliance, to set up optimal exercise programme, to
assess the effects of training on active muscle, on the myocardium
and on risk factors such as lipids, adrenergic system, fibrinolysis,
etc. The use of nuclear cardiology to approach some of these
problems was stressed recently, but we should avoid as much as
possible the introduction of sophisticated methods, principally for
the current practice.

     The evaluation of a rehabilitaiton programme is in fact not
easy, a large series of cases are required, with a good randomization,
a long term follow up and a critical discrimination of the
individual results. An example of these difficulties is given by
the study organized by the European Office of WHO (8), with the
collaboration of 24 centers and a total of 2.772 cases randomized
into two groups and a follow up of three years; the results will
be available only in 1980, but the interpretation of the results
will be diffucult : on one side, their is a poor compliance of
the intervention group and sometimes an incomplete programme, on
the other side a drop in cases and changes, during the year of the
study, of the attitudes of physicians and patients.

PSYCHOLOGICAL AND SOCIAL ASPECTS OF REHABILITATION

     At all stages of rehabilitation, the psychological and social
problems are of tremendous importance (9). Here again there are
many discussions on the methods used to assess psychological factors
and on the methods of treatment. Further investigations are needed
in this field. A good proof of the importance of psychosocial
factors is given by the study on patients after bypass surgery (10).

     It was demonstrated that the return to work after surgery
and improvement of the patient remains abnormally low; it is
related, not to the clinical or physiological situation, but

only to psychological and social factors.

We should also remember that the psychological approach should not be limited only to the patient, but should also be directed to the family and the employers.

SECONDARY PREVENTION AFTER MYOCARDIAL INFARCTION

Secondary prevention is the most recent part of the rehabilitation programme, but up to now its terms and conditions are not really too well defined. The correction of some risk factors (cigarette smoking, lipids abnormalities, hypertension, obesity), is probably important, but we don't know exactly what are these which are the most important. We don't know the exact influence of the prescription of drugs such as beta-blockers, Anturan, Aspirine, antiplatelets agents, etc. on the evolution or prognosis of a myocardial infarction. Further investigation in the secondary prevention is imperative and urgent (11,12).

ORGANIZATION OF CARDIAC REHABILITATION

Finally, the optimal organisation of rehabilitation remains an open question : should it be completely free (the patient returning home with adequate instruction for himself and for his practitioner), or institutionalized (the patient staying in a special institution for several weeks), or semi-institutionalized (the patient coming back to a special center 2 to 3 times a week for supervision and training). Very few data are available comparing the different systems, and probably these systems are more likely related to local habits and socio-cultural differences rather than to scientific arguments (13). Nevertheless it might be assumed that the necessity exists for health authorities to look into the problem, making available for doctors and patients the infrastructures needed for rehabilitation.

CONCLUSION

Important changes toward the approach of myocardial infarction have occurred during the last two decades. The immobilization of at least six weeks or more in all cases, with the consequence of an often permanent professional disablement is far behind us. It is generally agreed that earlier mobilization, physical exercise, functional evaluation, psycho-social approach, return to professional activity and secondary prevention are useful. But for all these attitudes, better information is required to evaluate the level of action and the new approaches should be based as much as possible on scientific and experimental data.

As a matter of fact, the current attitudes have modified the perspectives of our patients, even if it is not ascertained that their life expectancy is improved.

A permanent critical evaluation of the accepted recommendations, or of more recent recommendations is required (14).

We should not forget some basic principles: that physical activity is only a part of cardiac rehabilitation, and not always the more important; that technology should not be a limiting factor for implementation of cardiac rehabilitation, that more research is needed in all the fields of cardiac rehabilitation; that a better information of patients, doctors and health authority is needed.

Finally, we should show more interest on rehabilitation in other forms of cardio-vascular diseases, such as congenital or valvular diseases, operated or not, hypertension, etc.

References

1. Myocardial Infarction Community registers. WHO, Regional Office for Europe. Public Health in Europe. 5. (1976).
2. R. I. Levy. Progress in prevention of cardiovascular disease. Preventive Medicine. 7:464 (1978).
3. The rehabilitation of patients with cardiovascular diseases. WHO Regional Office for Europe. EURO 0381 (1969).
4. S. A. Levine and B. Lown. Armchair treatment of acute coronary thrombosis. J.Am.Med.Ass. 148:1365 (1952).
5. N. K. Wenger. Early ambulation after myocardial infarction: rationale, programme components and results in N. K. Wenger and H. Hellerstein. Rehabilitation of the coronary patient. J. Wiley and Sons, New York, (1978).
6. H. Denolin, M. Hoylaerts, C. De Lanthsheer, S. Degre and R. Bernard. Le test d'exercice précoce après infarctus du myocarde. Ann.Cardiol. Angeiol. 28:223 (1979).
7. J. A. Bonanno,. Coronary risk factor modification by chronic physical exercise, in E. A. Amsterdam, J. G. Wilmore and A. N. De Maria : Yorke Medical Book, New York (1977).
8. G. Lamm and D. L. Dorossiev. WHO Collaboration study on rehabilitation and comprehensive secondary prevention of patient after acute myocardial infarction, in: Advances in Cardiology, vol. 24, p.179. Karger, Basel, (1978).
9. E. L. Cay. Psychological approach in patients after a myocardial infarction, in: Advances in Cardiology, vol. 24, p.120. Karger, Basel, (1978).
10. P. David, H. Tenaille, M. Blain et H. Tremblay. Etude sur les facteurs de non retour au travail chez des cardiaques opérés. Union Médicale du Canada 105:1199 (1976).

11.   D. Elmfeldt, L. Wilhelmsen, I Vedin, C. Wilhelmsson, A.
      Hjalmarson and R. Bergstrand. General aspect of secondary
      prevention after myocardial infarction, in: Advances in
      Cardiology, vol. 24, p.94. Karger, Basel (1978).
12.   H. Blackburn. The potential for preventing reinfarction,
      in N. K. Wenger and H. Hellerstein, Rehabilitation of the
      Coronary patient. J. Wiley and Sons, New York (1978).
13.   J. Kallio. Results of rehabilitaiton in coronary patients,
      in Advances in Cardiology, vol. 24, p.153. Karger, Basel (1978).
14.   J. J. Kellermann and H. Denolin. Critical evaluation of
      cardiac rehabilitation. Bioliotheca Cardiologica. Vol.36.
      Karger, Basel.

CONTROVERSIES IN REHABILITATION OF THE

ISCHEMIC HEART DISEASE

V. Rulli

Centro per le Malattie Cardiovascolari
Ospedale S. Camillo
Rome, Italy

The analysis of results, procedures and methods utilised in the studies carried out from the end of the sixties until today on the rehabilitation of the IHD justify the stimulating and at the same time provocative title of this report: controversies in cardiac rehabilitation; ever since this term, so ill adjusted for the definition of a complex system of therapeutic interventions, entered the cardiological discipline, no congress, symposium or round table has taken place in which disputes have not emerged, throwing light and shade on the methods used and times and results achieved.

If this is due to the objective difficulties of the problem and the fragility of the material on which rehabilitation is required to operate, I think lack of information, improvisation and uncontrolled enthusiasm may also have contributed to the confusion.

When talking about controversies in rehabilitation, one presumes a complete separation from valuations that are not founded on acquired facts and which leave no space for interpretations that are no more than such. The quantity of data available even today is not enormous, but it is enough for a critical review; the rehabilitation of the ischemic heart disease is by now widely practiced all over the world, and in our country has constituted a real and important fact for some time.

I will recall only three international studies underway in the world: in the United States the National Exercise and Heart Disease Project, which involves six American centres, the W.H.O. "Evaluation of Comprehensive Rehabilitation and Preventive Programme for Patients

after Myocardial Infarction" and Götenborg's study and numerous
other minor projects some of which are even underway in the
developing countries.

These involve cooperative, long term studies which several
countries have been asked to collaborate in; this type of co-
operative research as Blackburn pointed out (1) constitutes the
big chance for medico-biological progress; but it presents
particular difficulty and high cost, as well as requiring great
caution in the elaboration and valuation: the randomised choice
of the material to study is difficult, as this can vary according to
the local socio-economic conditions;for the same reasons the
application of correct and standardised methodiologies which were
agreed upon in the programming phase, is not easy.

All the same, in spite of the serious difficulties that we
ourselves experienced in participating in one of these projects,
the advantages of the availability of a very high number of case
studies is undeniable and enables one to glimpse at the tendencies
of the phenomenon that one has decided to study, always on the
condition of saying "what you know and knowing what you are talking
about".

The postulate on which rehabilitation is based is that physical
activity can modify the development of ischemic heart disease:
it is a concept that has been derived by epidemiological research
and by attempts of primary prevention. In this sense rehabilitation
could not be other than the corollary of such a postulate.

There is general agreement on the fact that physical activity
has a favourable role in the health of man, given that it is such
an important part of his natural heredity; what is less easy to
accept is that physical activity,essential for the maintenance of
structural and functional integrity of skeletal muscle, can be
just as efficacious in the protection of the myocardium and his
vascular structure; as it is not easy to accept "tout court"
that an organ that functions more efficiently can function for a
longer period, or that once it has been damaged, it is less
inefficient.

I believe that these are the key points of our argument, about
which a series of misunderstandings have developed. Misunderstandings
which are also due to the fact that physical activity has been,
and is still, often talked about without underlining the fact that
only vigourous physical exercise can ever interfere in the incidence
of ischemic heart disease.

These are misunderstandings which, if on the one hand they
have disturbed the results of primary prevention, they have

contributed on the other, to the dispersion and to the impossibility of utilising many data which some co-operative studies were supposed to obtain.

The fact that many of the results available about the problem of the relationship between physical activity and ischemic heart disease have been obtained from different populations, as also occurs in the subject of rehabilitation, has complicated and will further complicate the possibility of discrimination, to the point where some authors have warned us against comparing "the apples with the pears", and from maintaining that a relationship of "cause and effect" has been acquired when we are merely dealing with association of effects.

On the other hand the controversies that divided by 1960 the participants in the Princeton Conference and at Makarska in 1963 and at Helsinki in 1967 showed themselves more recently in November 1977 at Luxembourg at the international conference on Physical Activity in the primary prevention of ischemic heart disease.

Admitted that physical activity may have a favourable effect on the prevention of ischemic heart disease and in the prevention of relapses, we need to define the mechanisms. If some of the physiological effects of physical activity are in fact well known, others remain arguable or unknown; those for example on the risk factors, cholesterol and triglycerides, arterial pressure, cutting down on smoking, variations of hemocoagulation, reduction of uricemia, etc. However, in spite of the series of interogatives that oppose the definitive clearing of the problem of primary prevention I believe that one can affirm with caution that in the field of secondary prevention and rehabilitation, things are perhaps a little clearer.

The fundemental points that I wish to discuss here are among the most controversial:
- the duration of mobilization after infarction, a problem that amalgamates with that of early rehabilitation and of early functional evaluation;
- training programmes and their psychological and physiological effects;
- the problems of the prognosis, morbidity and mortality and finally
- institutionalization of rehabilitation.

I believe that with such a pattern it will be easy to agree on which aspects of rehabilitation must be considered important and those which are less so.

   Since Samuel Levine's time in Boston when a patient was
confined, immobilized, to bed for six weeks after an acute
myocardial infarction up until today, the duration of the
immobilisation has been notably diminished, particularly for
those patients who have a non-complicated infarction. This
automatically coincided with the diffusion of the concept and
practice of early physical activation, deambulation and an early
return to work for throughly selected patients.

   The deleterious effects of prolonged immobilization (which
are too well known to be underlined here) go from hypovolemia to
the negativization of the nitrogen balance, from the reduction of
the contractile force of the skeletal muscle to psychological
problems of depression and anxiety.

   It has been widely enough demonstrated that the early
mobilization (within 8 to 15 days) of a patient with a non
complicated myocardial infarction is feasible and s fficiently safe
and that in selected patients morbidity and mortality are collocated
by similar values as in the groups of patients under control.

   Many problems, however, remain unclear: to what extent are
the effects of deconditioning deleterious after prolonged
hospitalization? Are we dealing with real or potential risks?
Do programmes of early physical activity modify the long-term risks
of a infarctual relapse or of sudden death? Are they capable of
modifying the total mortality for ischemic heart disease?

   At the moment only short term data are available for giving
an answer to these questions, even though the thesis of accurately
controlled early mobilization is becoming ever more widely accepted
to the point of actually constituting an integral part of treatment
in many countries throughout the world. Among the most interesting
data in this respect are those of Bloch(2), Harpur(3), Hayes(4),
Rose(5) and Hutter(6).

   McNeer's(7) retrospective study on 522 patients, and that of
Boyle(8) on 275 are even more important.

   Patients in convalescence for a myocardial infarction are
subject to an increased risk of death from cardiac causes in the
successive months and years, but early mobilization of non
complicated patients does not seem to raise such a risk.

   Boyle's study is important because it enumerates the conditions
that on the contrary oblige one to put off mobilization; the
presence of sinusal tachycardia which lasts for at least an hour
during the first 48 hours of hospitalization, the persistence
of depression equal or greater than 2 mm of the ST segment for six

days after the infarction, persistence of pain for 48 hours after
hospitalization, presence and persistence of some arrhythmias,
early multifocal ventricular premature beats, ventricular tachycardia,
ventricular fibrillation, a-v block of 2nd and 3rd degree, bundle
branch block.

We did not find differences in a group of non complicated
patients, mobilized between the 12th and 16th day from the acute
episode, and in a group mobilized between the 25th and 28th day
whatever the level of physical exercise before infarction, whatever
localisation of infarction, in the incidence of complications in
the two months following the beginning of observation.

Groden(9) in Glasgow found no difference in complications in a
study on two groups of patients mobilized respectively on the 15th
and 25th day.

In Boston, in Finland and in some English centres patients are
mobilized and made to walk three or even two days after an acute
episode.

These terms seem however rather excessive when one remembers
that anatomopathologists talk of 6 weeks for the formation of a
solid scar, and if one looks at White and Jetter's(10) research which
describes the highest incidence of heart rupture in mentally ill
people with infarction and not complying with immobility prescribed
by doctors.

It seems to me that many points remain to be cleared up as
far as early mobilization is concerned, in particular as regards the
real physiological advantages, that at long term and economic
advantages in the field of ischemic heart disease. I believe that
serious, prospective, randomised studies are still lacking, but that
above all we lack a serious classification of the patients condition,
classifications that should take numerous elements into account, the
site and nature of the infarction, enzymes, arterial pressure,
drugs, pulmonary pressure etc. all of which elements have a high
value in prediction, and which clinical observation is unable to
measure in other than a rough and ready manner.

On the other hand there is considerable disagreement on the
meaning of early mobilization; is it within the first week? within
the second?

The programme of early mobilization must always, in every case,
be associated with a comprehensive programme of psychological and
therapeutic support.

As far as the socio-economic aspects of the problem are concerned,
it seems to me that a return to work should be correlated with present

general working conditions rather than with programmes of early
rehabilitation. I do not feel that an early return to work is
fundamental to deduce, at least for the present and in the next
few years, the real advantages from early mobilisation with enough
statistical weight.

In the last few years, in addition to the concept of early
mobilisation, we have seen the association of the concept of making
the patient undergo (if he is without contra indications) an
early exercise test, 10 to 15 days after an acute episode and even
earlier in some centres. I feel that there has been a misunder-
standing also to this effect.

Making a patient undergo an early test of physical exercise
does not mean carrying out a maximal test and does not therefore
mean "sensu strictiori" practicing an ergometric test. If a test
does not measure the functional capacity of the subject at submaximal levels, it will be useful only to show up little else than
his ability to react to often unusual stimuli which may remain below
the threshold which trigger off phenomena which we wrongly thought
we could bring about by putting the patient on a cicloergometer and
making him pedal at 50-70 Watts, or at heart rate of 120/min. What
do these sort of tests propose at this moment? The observation of
the patients behaviour to enable one to prescribe the nature of the
activity that he can carry out in the period between discharge and
the beginning of active rehabilitation in the laboratory or in
sanatorium. Apart from the fact that a single test can only with
difficulty give satisfying results, and that the result is largely
conditioned by the level of capacity pre-existent to the infarction,
I maintain that it is preferable in this moment dynamic Holter
monitoring during which the patient is effectively studied during his
first days out of bed or the utilisation of telemetry during the first
days of mobilization. Thus one would avoid anxiety creating
situations which do little else than interfere with the results of
the trials.

We are not dealing here with the problem of risks: many studies
have now proved that early physical tests may not be damaging if
as long as contraindications are observed and as long as they are
of limited intensity even if the contraindications sometimes
present themselves beyond the limit of days chosen as being useful
for the execution of the trial.

That this can occur is shown by a very recent study by
Denolin(11) who carried out physical exercise tests on the tenth
day; of patients who had presented no problems during the test up
until a heart rate of 120, contraindications were found in 8 out
of 20 when rehabilitation was begun a month later.

We excluded 3 out of 18 patients who at the test carried out on the 15th day had not presented symptoms or signs of alarm and who at the beginning of laboratory rehabilitation 2 of whom showed instead manifest signs of left ventricular insufficiency and the third unstable angina.

J. P. Broustet(12) who has been very occupied with this problem said that to start training in the absence of signs or symptoms, it is sufficient to take the patient up to a frequency of 150/min., a month after the acute episode.

Kohn practices submaximal tests at the earliest after 30 days. In synthesis as regards this problem I would associate myself with those who maintain non-damaging and feasible an early physical exercise test before the 15th day and those who practice it for research reasons and with all the necessary precautions, but I would disassociate myself from those who maintain that it is indispensable or merely useful, and in every case I would disassociate myself decidedly from those who recommend it.

The notable variety of the different programmes of physical training has rendered definitive conclusions in many co-operative studies difficult.

In a recent study(14) it was ascertained that in 44 centres in 22 countries there was no common methodological standardization, not were there common lines for the selection of patients, nor common limits for ergometric tests.

The maximum heart rate that is reached in the preliminary tests before rehabilitation varies widely in the 44 centres within the groups of patients of the same age: in the age group 41-50 years the heart rate reached and varied between 120 and 187 beats per minute and in the successive age group between 110 and 179 beats per minute.

As far as indications for rehabilitation are concerned we know that in some centres the contraindications have not varied for five years and are as profoundly different as are their rehabilitation treatment methods; different to such an extent that no comparative elaboration is possible.

I do not believe that an ideal method of rehabilitation exists. It the aim of rehabilitation is to improve the quality of life, every patient who survives an infarction must be rehabilitated; he must be rehabilitated individually with methods and types of rehabilitation which may differ.

However, although the methods may differ, the principles of rehabilitation must be standardised without putting it off,

with continuity and globality in the sense that the psychological
and social factors must be held to be just as important as physical
exercise and training. It seems necessary to me to underline this
aspect given that many cardiologists still identify rehabilitation
with physical activity, overestimating its physiological effects.
A correct programme of rehabilitation includes three aspects; the
physiological one seen as a compensation for the irrepairable
consequence of the disease, the psychological one seen as the
reacquisition of self confidence and the secondary prevention.

The non-consideration of all these assumptions constitutes one
of the biggest shadows on rehabilitation.

Comprehensive programmes under three aspects could be started,
in agreement with local differences, both traditional and cultural,
both on an out-patient basis and in rehabilitation Centres for
controlled rehabilitation.

The number of patients with myocardial infarction is important,
and besides an ever bigger number of patients in an advanced stage
of illness can still gain some advantage from rehabilitation
methods. These facts underline the problem of cost and that of the
delayed return to work which may be brought about by rehabilitation
in sanatorium.

Certainly the difficulty in modifying many patient's life
style requires a notable educative activity which is more easily
realisable in rehabilitation Centres than in the out-patients
centres of a general hospital.

In West Germany and a few central European countries and in our
country there are sanatoria for rehabilitation. Their existence
seem justified by diagnostic, socio-therapeutic, educative and
curative arguments in the sense that a big centre guarantees a
rehabilitation based on diagnostic data that cannot be obtained in
out-patients, that psychological reconditioning and resocialization
are easier, and that it is possible to obtain more data to
establish a more accurate prognosis.

I feel personally that this sort of institutionalised
rehabilitation is too costly, that it prolongs the period before
return to work which early mobilization tries to limit, and that
it is only useful for a small number of patients. I think besides,
that it is favourable to let the patient free as soon as possible,
of course in relation to his condition. It is an advantage for the
patient to free himself as soon as possible from the awe of the
doctor, and that he does not become isolated from his family
environment; the sanatorium as one can notice in several studies,
reinforces the role of the illness, reduces indepedance and self
confidence and conditions loss of motivation.

On the other hand, even for those patients who flow to a centre where there is a functional evaluation unit, and where all diagnostic methods are possible, a rehabilitation that lasts as long as necessary is feasable at the necessary is feasable at the necessary level and which permits an adequate control of the patient.

As far as the physiological and psychological effects of rehabililitation are concerned I think that it is very important to answer the problem in the most honest and clearest way possible. Is physical training active in the sense of secondary prevention? The answer cannot be other than affirmative in the restrictive sense of the definition of coronary heart disease; on the other hand there are no data which sustain the idea that physical training is capable of modifying arteriosclerotic run-down of the coronary vessels. From this one deduces that adequate and regular physical activity may constitute an important part in a global rehabilitation project, as it has been proved that training improves cardiovascular functions and aerobic capacity.

A controversial point is whether the development of coronary collateral circulation is helped by training: this does not seem to be one of the secure advantages of rehabilitation, at least as regards our present knowledge.

A general agreement of the psychological effects of rehabilitation is not a difficult problem; more difficult and controversial however is the psychological or psychiatric intervention that must be carried out on the patient with psychological complications, also because from what has been said and done up until now, it seems that the psychologist or psychiatrist have been much more useful in satisfying the necessities of the cardiologist unable to face a difficult situation rather than necessities of the patient.(15)

If to quantify the effects of the psychological intervention is difficult, it is generally admitted that such effect are present and perhaps more lasting than the physiological effects. There do not seem to be reasonable doubts or controversies on this problem.

Let us move to the most controversial and discussed aspect of rehabilitation: its influence on morbidity and mortality.

Blackburn(16) affirmed recently that "the possibilities of a statistical analysis of the effects of rehabilitation on morbidity and mortality are rather modest given that the number of subjects studied is too scarse to affirm with certainty the efficiency of rehabilitation in this sense". We can add that not only is the number scarse but that the ways of treatment have differed, with the more or less prolonged duration and

contamination more or less important between treated subjects and
control subjects.

Randomized studies exist however, in which rehabilitation
constitutes the only method.

In one of these studies, Hakkila's(17), one sees a lesser
mortality within a year for a group of rehabilitated patients while
in the second year of observation such differences in mortality
between those rehabilitated and those of control group diminished.
The author concludes that the effect of the intervention on mortality
seem modest, especially when one sets apart the data of mortality
within a year.

In Sanne's(18) study over four years of observation there was
a mortality of 17% in the group of patients under treatment,
and of 22% in control patients; coronary mortality was 14% and 21%
respectively in the patients in control without significant
differences as regards the cause, the type or site of death in the
control group and experimental group.

Stratifying the patients according to the different types of
risks of new fatal events by means of a logistic analysis, Sanne
observed a lesser mortality in those rehabilitated than in those non
rehabilitated. The difference nevertheless was not significant from
a statistical point of view. In the group of subjects under treatment the patients who remained closest to the programme had a lesser
mortality, but these already presented at the beginning a lesser
risk of cardiac death.

As far as regards infarctual relapses Sanne was unable to
observe differences between the two groups those under treatment
and those under control. This study too, interesting as it is, is
criticizable for the number of drop outs in the training course and
for the importance of the numerous demotivying factors which Sanne
himself referred to.

Other authors have obtained data that only show a tendency
towards a lower mortality in treated patients. However, in these
studies the randomization was not correct. After having considered
such data we must recognize that for numerous reasons further,
well controlled studies are necessary for answering the fundamental
question whether or not rehabilitation modifies morbidity and
mortality. It does not therefore seem to me that in the present
state one can honestly justify rehabilitation only on the basis of
a secure interference of the treatment on morbidity and mortality.

What then are the reasons for which we feel ourselves so
envolved in the rehabilitation of our patients?

Undoubtedly to satisfy the aspects which are cited in its
definition: improve the patients physiological condition, re-
construct him psychologically, recondition his social status in a
society where work is synonymous with sociality, and to try, ever
within the limits of our knowledge and against objective
difficulties, not only in the research field but perhaps also in
the biological one, to improve our prognosis. These are the aims
of rehabilitation, this its' meaning in spite of the light and
shadow that I have attempted to outline here.

References

1. H. Blackburn, Coronary risk factors. How to evaluate and
    manage them. Europ. J. Cardiol. 23:249 (1975).
2. A. Block, J. P. Maeder, J. C. Haissly, J. Felix and J.
    Blackburn, Early mobilisation after myocardial infarction.
    A controlled study. Am. J. Cardiol. 34:151 (1974).
3. J. E. Harpur, W. T. Conner, M. Hamilton, R. J. Keller,
    H. I. B. Galbraith, J. J. Murray and G. A. Rose, Controlled
    trial of early mobilisation and discharge from the hospital
    in uncomplicated myocardial infarction. Lancet 2:1331 (1971).
4. M. J. Hayes, U. R. Morris and J. R. Hampton, Comparison of
    two and nine day mobilisation in patients admitted to hospital
    with myocardial infarction. Brit. Ht. J. 36:395 (1974).
5. G. Rose, Early mobilisation and discharge after myocardial
    infarction. Modern Concepts of cv. Disease 12:59 (1972).
6. A. M. Hutter, V. W. Sidel, K. J. Shine and R. W. de Santis,
    Early hospital discharge after myocardial infarction, New
    England J. Med. 288:1141 (1973).
7. J. F. McNeer, A. G. Wallace, G. S. Wagner, C. F. Stramer and
    R. A. Rosati, The course of acute myocardial infarction.
    Feasibility of early discharge of uncomplicated patients,
    Circulation 51:410 (1975).
8. M. L. Boyle, J. M. Barber, G. Shivalingappa, M. J. Walsh and
    N. C. Chaturvedi, Early mobilisation and discharge of patients
    with acute myocardial infarction, Lancet 2:57 (1972).
9. R. M. Groden, The management of myocardial infarction, A
    controlled study of the effects of early mobilisation, Card.
    Rehab. 1:13 (1971).
10. W. Jetter and P. D. White, Rupture of the heart in patients
    in mental institutions, Am. Ht. J. 21:783 (1944).
11. H. Denolin, Unpublished data,(1978).
12. J. P. Broustet, La Readaptation des coronariens, Sandoz Ed.,
    Paris(1973).
13. R. M. Kohn, A critique to ambulation studies, Critical Eval.,
    of Card. Rehab. Biblthca cardiol n. 36 Karger, Basel (1977).
14. J. J. Kellermann, H. Denolin and K. Konig, Rehabilitation
    methodology, international survey, Critical Eval. of Card.
    Rehab. in Biblthca cardiol.n.36 Karger, Basel (1977).

15.   T. Strasser, Introduction Panel III in Critical Eval. of
      Card. Rehab., Biblthca cardiol. n. 36 Karger, Basel (1977).
16.   H. Blackburn, Rehabilitation, Mortality and Morbidity in
      C.H.D. In. Critical Eval. of Card. Rehab., Biblthca cardiol.
      n.36 Karger, Basel (1977).
17.   J. Hakkila and O. Lucerila, Study in progress, Unpublished
      observations.
18.   H. Sanne, Physical training of the myocardial infarction, In
      Critical Eval. of Card. Rehab., Biblthca cardiol. n. 36
      Karger, Basel (1977).

EARLY MOBILIZATION AFTER MYOCARDIAL INFARCTION:

HISTORICAL PERSPECTIVE AND CRITICAL APPRAISAL

Nanette Kass Wenger

Emory University School of Medicine
Atlanta,
Georgia

INTRODUCTION

The current pattern of care for the patient with myocardial infarction, particularly the patient with an uncomplicated or minimally complicated clinical course, is characterized by an abbreviation of the period at bed rest, by a decrease in imposed activity restriction and invalidism with an earlier resumption of physical activity, and by earlier discharge from the hospital for appropriately selected individuals. Indeed, early ambulation and early hospital dismissal commonly go hand in hand, the former enabling the latter to occur.

This presentation will delineate the physiologic basis for early ambulation, summarize the data relating the the efficacy and safety of this approach, and present guidelines for patient selection and early ambulation implementation.

EARLY AMBULATION: PHYSIOLOGIC BASIS

The early empiric advocacy of physical activity by Heberden and by Parry as beneficial for the patient with angina pectoris was superseded, in the early 1900s, by a regimen of protracted and almost complete bed rest for the patient with myocardial infarction. The scientific basis was the Mallory-White-Salcedo-Salgar anatomic study of the healing of myocardial infarction; the investigators demonstrated that at least six weeks were required to transform necrotic myocardium into firm scar tissue and raised the fear that activity would increase the likelihood of dysrhythmia, aneurysm formation, myocardial rupture, or asystole and sudden cardiac death. We now realize that their findings described the myocardial

21

healing among the very ill post-infarction patients who
subsequently died, a status not necessarily comparable to that of
survivors. Current documentation identifies that survival is
uncommon among patients with massive left ventricular infarction,
a typical finding in their autopsy series, because of inadequate
residual pumping function, cardiac output and myocardial perfusion.
We also know that scar formation, the fibrous replacement of
necrotic myocardium, proceeds from the periphery and thus progresses
more rapidly to completion within a smaller area of infarction.
Among patients seen in Coronary Care Units today, these smaller
anatomic areas of infarction are characteristic, with the diagnosis
of myocardial infarction frequently based on serial ST-T electrocardiographic changes with or without cardiac serum enzyme
alterations; this is in contrast to the massive transmural (Q
wave) infarctions which fulfilled the criteria for diagnosis in
theMallory-White-Salcedo-Salgar study. Indeed, today, many patients
are considered to have myocardial infarction and managed accordingly
based solely on their chest pain history (with and without
angiographic confirmation of coronary obstructive disease), even
without other objective evidence of myocardial necrosis.

The current trend toward early mobilization was begun by Dr.
Samuel Levine of Boston in the 1940s; his "chair treatment of
coronary thrombosis" was based on the theory that the sitting
position increased peripheral venous pooling, decreased venous
return, and thus reduced cardiac work. Although no controlled
series was done, there were no complications of this regimen among
the 81 patients initially reported; Levine allowed his patients to
sit in a chair for one to two hours daily, beginning the first day
after myocardial infarction. He reasoned that this approach would
diminish thromboembolic and respiratory complications, a thesis that
has subsequently been well documented and accepted. Drs. Levine,
Dock and Harrison all warned that excessive physician caution
might result in incapactitating cardiac neurosis in post-infarction
patients, and that an enhanced sense of well-being and easier work
resumption accompanied liberalization of activity restriction.
Dock further recommended the use of a bedside commode rather than
a bedpan; it has subsequently been documented that cardiac output
and myocardial work decrease in the sitting as compared with the
recumbent position; thus less energy is required to use a bedside
commode than a bedpan. Indeed, there is no significant increase in
cardiac work, as estimated by the rate-pressure (heart rate times
systolic blood pressure), with the postural change and selected
low-level active and passive exercise commonly performed by patients
in early ambulation programmes in the Coronary Care Unit. Data
from the cardiac catheterization studies of Stead and associated
demonstrating the marked increase in cardiac output with fear and
anxiety, were the basis for suggesting that enforced bed rest might
exert a paradoxic effect, with the patient's fear of impending
death or disability or his concern about prolonged invalidism

resulting in increased cardiac work in response to emotional stress.

It was, nevertheless, specific physiologic information about the deleterious effect of prolonged immobilization at bed rest that provided the current impetus for early ambulation programmes for patients with myocardial infarction, as well as for patients after successful aortocoronary bypass surgery.

The most marked alteration seen with prolonged immobilization at bed rest is a decrease in physical work capacity. A study of healthy college students, placed at strict bed rest for 21 days, identified that their exercise test performance after immobilization was characterized by a 20 to 25 percent decrement in maximal oxygen uptake. At least three weeks of exercise training were required to restore the pre-bed rest physical work capacity; the greater the physical fitness prior to bed rest, the longer the period of re-training required to restore the pre-bed rest functional level. These data must be considered in evaluating the post-illness fatigue, weakness and asthenia of patients subjected to prolonged bed rest; do these symptoms reflect the disease or the management imposed for the illness?

When the patient is initially mobilized after an extended period at bed rest, both a moderate tachycardia and a decreased adapability to change in posture, postural hypotension occur, potentially adverse responses in a post-infaction patient. Although loss of normal postural vasomotor reflexes plays a role, the major etiologic factor is hypovolemia, as the circulating blood volume may decrease by as much as 700-800 cc after a week to ten days at bed rest. Of additonal concern with the bed-rest induced hypovolemia is that the plasma volume decreases to a greater extent than does the red blood cell mass, increasing blood viscosity and predisposing the patient to thromboembolic complications; this occurs in the setting where bed rest minimizes the use of the leg muscle pump adding the thromboembolic risk of venous circulatory stasis to that of increased blood viscosity.

A negative nitrogen and protein balance are encountered and may potentially adversely effect the healing of a necrotic area of myocardium. Pulmonary ventilation is diminished, due to a decrease in lung volume and vital capacity; this may be particularly important in the patient with associated chronic pulmonary disease.

Finally, there is a decrease of 10 to 15 percent in muscular contractile strength after a week at bed rest, associated with a decrease in skeletal muscular mass. Inefficiently contracting muscle demands more oxygen for the performance of any particular activity and imposes this increased oxygen cost on a potentially ischemic myocardium.

In addition to lessening these "deconditioning" effects of prolonged immobilization, early ambulation is also warranted to decrease the anxiety and depression which accompany, although to a varying extent, most episodes of acute myocardial infarction, because most psychotropic drugs are contraindicated for the patient with symptomatic coronary atherosclerotic heart disease due to their adverse effects on heart rate, blood pressure and cardiac rhythm, the benefical effect of physical activity is of particular value. The gradually progressive increase in activity permitted each day affords the post-infarction patient tangible evidence of improvement, alaying the anxiety and depression response and reinforcing the physician's assertion that the patient may expect to return to a normal or near-normal lifestyle.

STUDIES OF EARLY AMBULATION: SAFETY AND EFFICACY

A number of the initial nonrandomized descriptive studies of early ambulation in a variety of populations uniformly suggested a favourable outcome: improved ability to perform self-care and usual household tasks, enhanced self-image and emotional outlook, earlier discharge from the hospital, and a more optimal return to work and/ or to pre-illness lifestyle. Indeed, long-term follow-up data identified no differences in outcome as the period at bed rest and the duration of hospitalization were decreased.

The Duke Medical Centre study, surveying 522 consecutive patients with myocardial infarctions, found that none of the 51% with an uncomplicated clinical course through day 4 had subsequent hospital mortality or late complications. They recommended that this patient group be considered for early mobilization and early hospital discharge.

A number of randomized clinical trials have subsequently yielded comparable data; it must, however, be emphasized that the time of early mobilization in the earlier studies is often comparable to the time of late mobilization (conventional therapy) in more recent series. Also, criteria for the diagnosis of myocardial infarction varied considerably as did the designation of a complicated or uncomplicated clinical course and the time during the hospitalization at which this decision was made; furthermore, many trials involved small numbers of patients. Therefore, it is inappropriate to group the data from the several trials and preferable to examine each individually.

Groden and Brown's study compared patients mobilized on day 14 and discharged on day 21 with those managed in the traditional manner with mobilization on day 25 and discharge on day 35. The early ambulation group was characterized by a lower neuroticism score at the time of hospital discharge; however, at the one-year re-examination there was no difference in psychologic test scores, suggesting that the initial advantage of the rehabilitative approach during the hospitalization may be lost if this is not continued in the post-hospital phase. In a subsequent study, Groden noted fewer psychologic complications and an earlier return to work among patients mobilized on day 15 and discharged on day 22, as compared with a control group mobilized on day 25 and sent home by day 36; no adverse effects of early ambulation were apparent.

The British study of Harper et al., in an 8-month follow-up, showed no difference in morbidity and mortality between patients mobilized on day 8 and discharged on day 15 and those who remained at bed rest for 21 days and were hospitalized for a total duration of 28 days; there was an earlier return to work in the early ambulation group. Lamers and associates in the Netherlands defined that mobilization on day 9 and discharge at 3 weeks was safe for patients with an uncomplicated clinical course; at 1 1/2 years of follow-up there was no difference in the clinical course of the illness.

The Boston study of Hutter et al., comparing patients discharged at 2 weeks with those discharged at 3 weeks, showed no differences at 6 months of follow-up; the investigators concluded that the additional week of hospitalization afforded no benefit and that the abbreviated hospital stay permitted an economy in cost and in hospital bed utilization. Comparable data are available from the study of Boyle and Lorimer comparing large numbers of patients discharged at 3 and 4 weeks respectively.

Hayes' evaluation of uncomplicated myocardial infarction patients discharged at day 9 and day 16 respectively showed no discernible difference in morbidity and mortality. In the Geneva trial of Block et al., patients mobilized at day 2-3 and discharged by day 21 were compared with a control group mobilized on day 21 and hospitalized for a mean duration of 33 days. Morbidity, mortality, and exercise test results were comparable at one year of follow-up, but the early mobilization group had less disability and an earlier return to work; importantly, psychologic factors constituted the main determinants of disability.

Based on these and other studies, the safety of supervised early mobilization appears established for appropriately selected patients with myocardial infarction. This pattern of care has not been associated with an increase in in-hospital or follow-up complications: angina pectoris, recurrent myocardial infarction, dysrhythmias, congestive heart failure, ventricular aneurysm, cardiac rupture, sudden cardiac death, etc.; indeed, some studies suggested a more favourable outcome. The benefits of early ambulation include a reduction of the complications of prolonged immobilization at bed rest; thromboembolism, pulmonary atelectasis, cardiovascular deconditioning, anxiety, depression and dependency. At the time of discharge, early ambulation patients have an improved

functional capacity, and a follow-up examination there is greater
disability with the traditional hospital regimen. The early
mobilization group is also characterized by an earlier and more
complete return to work.

PATIENT SELECTION AND PROGRAMME COMPONENTS

The appropriate selection of patients is an essential feature
in assuring the safety and benefit of early ambulation. Early
ambulation may begin as early as the initial days in the Coronary
Care Unit for the patient with an uncomplicated clinical course,
defined as an individual without significant shock, congestive
heart failure, dysrhythmia, or persistent or recurrent chest pain.
Patients with these complications require specific management at
bed rest, and ambulation should be deferred until the complications
have been controlled. Nevertheless, this uncomplicated patient
group constitutes almost half of all patients admitted to Coronary
Care Units in the U.S.; in general, they tend to be younger persons
and those with an initial episode of myocardial infarction, i.e.
patients with a more favourable outlook.

The general principles for early ambulation are that the
activities should be low-level in intensity, be gradually progressive,
be isotonic rather than isometric, and be supervised by an individual
trained to evaluate the physiologic response to the level of activity.
Isotonic (dynamic or aerobic) activities elicit a heart rate response
proportional to the intensity of the activity; heart rate response
may therefore be used to monitor the gradually progressive activity
increments. Isometric exercise by contrast, may elicit a
precipitous increase in blood pressure proportional to the percent
of maximum voluntary contraction of the muscle group; this increased
afterload is potentially poorly tolerated by an ischemic left
ventricle and may result in pain and/or life-threatening dysrhythmia.
Isometric activity should be avoided early in the clinical course of
myocardial infarction and limited in the subsequent management of
patients with symptomatic coronary atherosclerotic heart disease.

A prototype early ambulation programme, employed at Grady
Memorial Hospital and the Emory University School of Medicine in
Atlanta, Georgia since the mid 1960s, is incorporated into the
comprehensive plan of care for patients with myocardial infarction.
Fourteen serial activity steps include parallel intensities of
prescribed exercise, in-hospital daily living activities, and
recreational-educational-diversional activities. During the
early years of our programme, when the myocardial infarction patient
with an uncomplicated clinical course was typically hospitalized
for 16-21 days, patients customarily advanced one step each day.
As the hospitalization for patients with uncomplicated myocardial
infarction has become progressively abbreviated, we have retained
our 14 step format, but typically allow the patient to accomplish
two steps each day. The advantage of this approach is that the more
gradual, detailed activity progression can be employed for the more

impaired patients, the ones with a previously complicated hospital course, those for whom the duration of hospitalization tends to be longer.

Activity surveillance, both in the Coronary Care Unit and during the remainder of the hospitalization, includes identification of inappropriate responses to activity: (1) a heart rate response greater than 120/min., (2) chest pain, dyspnea, or excessive fatigue, (3) the occurence of dysrhythmia, (4) ST segment displacement on the electrocardiogram or monitor as evidence of ischemia, and (5) a decrease of greater than 15-20 mm Hg in systolic blood pressure; the usual response to activity is a slight increase in systolic blood pressure, and, in the clinical setting, a fall in systolic blood pressure can be equated with inadequacy of the cardiac output to meet activity demand. The occurence of any of these inappropriate physiologic responses to low-level activity signifies that the workload is excessive and requires that the patient's activity plan be revised, that the patient be returned to a lower activity level and that the clinical status be carefully re-evaluated. When the response to early ambulation is appropriate, the patient may safely progress to the next activity level.

Coronary Care Unit low-level activities are in the range of 1-2 mets (1 to 2 times the resting metabolic rate; 1 met = approximately 3.5 ml O_2/kg body weight/minute). Activities include self-care, eating, the use of a bedside commode and sitting in bed or in a bedside chair for progressively increasing intervals. These activities entail little or no augmentation of myocardial oxygen demand. Isotonic active and passive arm and leg movements are performed, with the supervising nurse or therapist observing and recording the physiologic responses previously cited.

After the patient leaves the Coronary Care Unit, the goal of progressive physical activity is for the patient to attain a functional level which will enable self-care and usual household activities by the time of discharge from the hospital. This is currently as early as the 10th to 14th day for the patient with an uncomplicated clinical course. Details of physical activity programmes vary considerably, but fundamental principles are that they be low-level in intensity (2-3 mets), be supervised as previously described, be gradually progressive in work demand, and remain primarily isotonic in character. Low-intensity, rhythmic calisthenics are used to maintain muscle tone and joint mobility, but the major prescriptive activity is walking, gradually increasing the distance walked and the pace of walking, with the aim of increasing endurance. Ideally, physical activity is performed several times each day, interspersed with rest periods. It is desirable for patients who will have to climb stairs at home to do so before leaving the hospital, walking down a flight of stairs and returning by elevator one day, and walking slowly up a flight

of steps the next. Accomplishing this task safely in the hospital
allays the anxiety of both the patient and the family when stair-
climbing is initiated on return home.

There is advantage in a predefined activity programme for
early ambulation. It is unrealistic to expect physicians to write
detailed physical activity orders each day; even if this were
feasible, the considerable minimal physician-to-physician variations
in activity preference would make it difficult for a hospital staff
to implement the activities; finally it is reassuring to the patient
to know the anticipated activity progression in the absence of
complications. The Grady-Emory early ambulation patient record
protocol contains a column to be completed by the activity
supervisor who records the patient's heart rate, blood pressure,
and symptomatic response to each level of activity; the physician,
on the same protocol form, initials permission for the daily
progression from one activity level to the next. This format
enhances communication among personnel caring for the patient,
leading to improved patient care.

SUMMARY

Recent data increasingly confirm that most serious complications
of myocardial infarction occur during the initial days of hospitalization; the overwhelming majority of patients with an uncomplicated
clinical course during the first 3-4 days have little or no in-
hospital mortality and few serious late complications. These data
and information concerning the risks of needlessly prolonged
activity restriction have encouraged both early mobilization and
earlier discharge from the hospital for appropriately selected
post-infarction patients.

The safety of supervised early ambulation for appropriately
selected patients after an uncomplicated acute myocardial infarction
is no longer controversial. Benefits of early ambulation include
the prevention of deconditioning and other complications of
prolonged bed rest; a decrease in anxiety and depression, a greater
functional capacity and an improved self-image at the time of
hospital discharge; and the economic advantages of permitting a
shorter hospitalization, more optimal hospital bed utilization,
and an earlier and more complete return to work. Early ambulation
is a desirable, feasible, cost-effective and safe approach to
patient care.

References

1. J. Acker: Early ambulation of post-myocardial infarction patients. In: Naughton J.P., Hellerstein H. K. (eds.): "Exercise Testing and Exercise Training in Heart Disease." Academic Press, New York, (1973).
2. A. A. J. Adgey: Prognosis after early discharge from hospital of patients with acute myocardial infarction. Br Heart J. 31:730 (1969).
3. A. Bloch, J-P. Maeder, J-C. Haissly, et al: Early mobilization after myocardial infarction. A controlled study. Am J Cardiol 34: 152, (1974).
4. C. D. Bonner: Rehabilitation instead of bed rest? Geriatrics 24:109, (1969).
5. J. A. Boyle, A. R. Lorimer: Early mobilisation after uncomplicated myocardial infarction. Prospective study of 538 patients. Lancet 2:346, (1973).
6. J. P. Broustet, M. Dubecq, J. Bouloumie, et al: Rehabilitation of the coronary patients: Mobilization program in the acute phase. Schweiz Med Wochenschr 103:57, (1973).
7. P. Brummer, V. Kallio, E. Tala: Early ambulation in the treatment of myocardial infarction. Acta Med Scand 180:231, (1966).
8. N. H. Cassem, T. P. Hackett: Psychiatric consultation in a coronary care unit. Ann Intern Med 75:9, (1971).
9. N. C. Chaturvedi, M. J. Walsh, A. Evans, et al: Selection of patients for early discharge after acute myocardial infarction. Br Heart J., 36:533, (1974).
10. R. F. DeBusk, A. P. Spivack, A. van Kessell, et al: The coronary care unit activities program: Its role in post-infarction rehabilitation. J Chronic Dis., 24:373 (1971).
11. J. E. Deitrick, G. D. Whedon, E. Shorr: Effects of immobilization upon various metabolic and physiologic functions of normal men. Am J Med., 4:3, (1948).
12. W. Dock: The evil sequelae of complete bed rest. JAMA 125:1083, (1944).
13. M. Duke: Bed rest in acute myocardial infarction. A study of physician practices. Am Heart J., 82:486, (1971).
14. K. Fareeduddin, W. H. Abelmann: Impaired orthostatic tolerance after bed rest in patients with myocardial infarction. N Engl J Med 280:345, (1969).
15. B. M. Groden: The management of myocardial infarction. A Controlled study on the effects of early mobilization. Cardiac Rehabil., 1:13, (1971).
16. R. I. F. Brown: Differential psychological effects of early and late mobilization after myocardial infarction. Scan J Rehabil Med., 2:60, (1970).
17. J. E. Harpur, R. J. Kellett, W. T. Conner, et al: Controlled trial of early mobilization and discharge from hospital in uncomplicated myocardial infarction. Lancet 2:1331, (1971).

18. T. R. Harrison: Abuse of rest as a therapeutic measure for patients with cardiovascular disease. JAMA 125:1075, (1944).

19. M. J. Hayes, G. K. Morris, J. R. Hamptom: Comparison of mobilization after two and nine days in uncomplicated myocardial infarction. Br Med J., 3: 10, (1974).

20. A. M. Hutter Jr., V. W. Sidel, K. I. Shine, et al: Early hospital discharge after myocardial infarction. N Engl J Med., 288: 1141, (1973).

21. C. W. Irvin Jr., A. M. Burgess Jr.: The abuse of bed rest in the treatment of myocardial infarction. N Engl J Med., 243:486, (1950).

22. W. W. Jetter, P. D. White: Rupture of the heart in patients in mental institutions. Ann Intern Med., 21:783, (1944).

23. H. J. Lamers, W. S. J. Drost, B. J. M. Kroon, et al: Early mobilization after myocardial infarction: A controlled study. Br Med J., 1:257, (1973).

24. S. A. Levine: Some harmful effects of recumbency in the treatment of heart disease. JAMA, 126:80, (1944).

25. T. N. Lynch, R. L. Jensen, P. M. Stevens, et al: Metabolic effects of prolonged bed rest: Their modification by simulated altitude. Aerosp Med 38:10, (1967).

26. J. F. McNeer, G. S. Wagner, P. B. Ginsburg, et al: Hospital discharge one week after acute myocardial infarction. N Engl J Med., 298:229, (1978).

27. A. G. Wallace, G. S. Wagner, et al: The course of acute myocardial infarction. Feasibility of early discharge of the uncomplicated patient. Circulation, 51:410, (1975).

28. B. D. McPherson, A. Paivio, M. S. Yuhasz, et al: Psychological effects of an exercise program for post-infarct and normal adult men. J Sports Med Phys Fitness, 7:95, (1967).

29. G. K. Mallory, P. D. White, J. Salcedo-Salgar: The speed of healing of myocardial infarction: A study of the pathologic anatomy in seventy-two cases. Am Heart J 18:647, (1939).

30. P. B. Miller, R. L. Johnson, L. E. Lamb: Effects of moderate physical exercise during four weeks of bed rest on circulatory functions in man. Aerosp Med., 36:1077, (1965).

31. R. Mulcahy, N. Hickey: The rehabilitation of patients with coronary heart disease: A comparison of the return to work specific rehabilitation programme. J Ir Med Assoc., 64:541, (1971).

32. D. O. Nutter, R. C. Schlant, J. W. Hurst: Isometric exercise and the cardiovascular system. Mod Concepts Cardiovasc Dis., 41:11, (1972).

33. Report of the Joint Working Party of Royal College of Physicians of London and the British Cardiac Society on Rehabilitation after Cardiac Illness: Cardiac rehabilitation 1975. JR Coll Physicians Lond., 9:281, (1975).

34. Report of the Task Force on Cardiovascular Rehabilitation, National Heart and Lung Institute: Needs and Opportunities for Rehabilitating the Coronary Heart Disease Patient,

December 5, 1974. Washington, DC, US Department of Health, Education, and Welfare publication (NIH) 75-750.

35. G. Rose: Early mobilization and discharge after myocardial infarction. Mod Concepts Cardiovasc Dis., 41:59, (1972).

36. G. R. Royston: Short stay hospital treatment and rapid rehabilitation of cases of myocardial infarction in a district hospital. Br Heart J., 34:526, (1972).

37. B. Saltin, G. Blomqvist, J. H. Mitchell, et al: Response to exercise after bed rest and training. Circulation 37-38 (Suppl. 7): 1, (1968).

38. H. J. C. Swan, H. W. Blackburn, R. DeSanctis, et al: Duration of hospitalization in "uncomplicated completed acute myocardial infarction." An ad hoc committee review. Am J Cardiol, 37:413, (1976).

39. J. Takkunen, E. Huhti, O. Oilinki, et al: Early ambulation in myocardial infarction. Acta Med Scand 188:103, (1970).

40. H. H. Tucker, P. H. M. Carson, N. M. Base, et al: Results of early mobilization and discharge after myocardial infarction. Br Med J., 1:10, (1973).

41. J. Wanka: Bedpan vs. commode in patients with myocardial infarction. Cardiac Rehabil, 1:7, (1970).

42. N. K. Wenger: Coronary Care - Rehabilitation after Myocardial Infarction, prepared for the Coronary Care Committee, Council on Clinical Cardiology and the Committee on Medical Education, American Heart Association, Dallas, Texas EM609, November 1973.

43. H. K. Hellerstein, H. Blackburn, et al: Uncomplicated myocardial infarction. Current physician practice in patient management. JAMA 244:511, (1973).

EARLY EXERCISE TEST AFTER MYOCARDIAL INFARCTION AND IN

UNSTABLE ANGINA

J. P. Broustet, J. F. Cherrier, J. Hilaire, and P. Guern

Hôpital Cardiologique du Haut Leveque
Avenue de Magellan
33604 Pessac, France

INTRODUCTION

Acute myocardial infarction and unstable angina do result
in bed rest. In uncomplicated cases, the rapid relief of symptoms
allows early ambulation and earlier discharge.

Then arise question marks:

What are the risks for the next future?

When to start with physical training?

Has the proper choice of drugs been made?

What is the status of coronary bed in non infarcted
areas?

Early exercise test (EET) soon after myocardial infarction
or after control of pain in unstable angina may provide a valuable
contribution to these important questions.

The purposes of EET are the following:

1. Earlier detection of latent complications: Resting
    examination is a poor tool to predict the risk of
    sudden death, reinfarction, angina, especially in
    uncomplicated cases: exercise induced occurrence of
    chest pain, S-T segment changes, arrythmias will get
    the physician aware of such complications.

2.   Improvement and control of proper therapy: exercise
      test is a reproducible, safe, precise tool in evaluating,
      comparing the effect of drugs or of combinations of
      drugs. Here the objective is to discharge the patient
      with the best functional result and the minimum of
      risks especially after unstable angina.

3.   Increase of self confidence.

      When the results are good, the patient's hope of adequate
      recovery is reinforced. When they are poor, it is still
      easy at this stage to stress on the precocity of test,
      and its usefulness to find out the best therapy
      relying on new comparative exercise tests.

4.   Improvement of quality of physical training is due to
      earlier knowledge that many patients may have safe
      exercise sessions after 3 weeks. Thus reconditioning will
      start earlier and will be more safe and intensive in
      those patients who had uncomplicated early exercise test.

PROTOCOLE

     A routine exercise protocole used in the daily practice in
our laboratory applied well for this subgroup: exercise test
was performed on an electrically braked bicycle at a pedalling
speed of 60 rpm in upright position.

     The first stage was 30 watts. Every stage had a duration of
three minutes and an increment of 30 watts.

     Indeed the criteria for cessation of the test were slightly
less "hard":

     -   target heart rate was reduced at 90% of 220 minus age

     -   non isolated ventricular premature beats of bigeminism
         or more that   10% of QRS complexes.

     -   S-T segment depression greater than four mm in non
         infarcted area.

     Exercise ECG. Exercise lead system has been previously
described. We use routinely CM5 facing antero lateral wall,
ML5 postero diaphragmatic area and VE exploring anter-septal area.
We utilized the computerized system of Marquette designed for
exercise testing. Thus every QRS complex is the mean of twenty
five complexes after suppression of muscle noise, baseline shift,
alternative current and respiratory variations. After cessation
of exercise the printer provides a summary with the last twenty

five QRS complexes of every stage of three minutes and of every minute of recovery:

CM5 is located in the upper part

ML5 in the middle strip

VE in the lower strip

Moreover computer provides an histogram S-T segment depression and S-T slope for each of three leads.

The contra-indication to true early exercise test were as follows:

1. After myocardial infarction.

    a) Careful checking of the actual onset of infarction which may be more recent than impending infarction or unstable predictive angina leading to admission to coronary care unit.

    b) Feaver, pericardial rub, chest pain evoking aneurysm.

    c) Recent extension of M.I., or new ST-T changes with chest pain.

    d) Circulatory and X ray indications of resting cardiac failure.

    e) Major ST elevation in many chest leads.

    f) Non isolated extrasystoles.

    g) General contraindications: age over 70.

    h) Absence of early mobilization in or out of coronary care unit.

2. After unstable angina.

    1. A five days period without chest pain was the primary condition.

    2. In patients exhibiting large and extended S-T depressions with a mild acceleration of heart rate we did not wait until occurrence of chest pain. In other, chest pain, if any, was the criteria for cessation of test.

I - RESULTS IN MYOCARDIAL INFARCTION

We divided early exercise tests after M.I. into two subgroups:

First: true early exercise test performed before primary
discharge (fifteenth to twentieth day in uncomplicated cases).

Secondly: delayed early exercise test: the test was
delayed because they were apparent contra-indication to true
early test: such as large infarction or angina when walking on
the level or persistance of S-T segment elevation in many leads.
In those patients bi-dimensional echocardiography was done and
if the kinetics of left ventricule was severely reduced in a
large area exercise test was not performed.

They were thirteen males and two females aged from thirty
to sixty eight years (table 1).

Infarctions were located in various areas.

TABLE 1

```
┌─────────────────────────────────────────────────────────────┐
│                    EARLY EXERCISE TEST                        │
│                                                               │
│               POST MYOCARDIAL INFARCTION                      │
│                                                               │
│            (Before day 20 th : mean : day 16th)               │
│         15pts : 13M, 2W-AGE 53 ± 10 years (30 →68)            │
│                          Antero-septal........... 3           │
│                          Anterior ............... 3           │
│         M.I. location    Postero-lateral ........ 3           │
│                          Postero-apical ......... 1           │
│                          Postero-basal .......... 4           │
│                                                               │
└─────────────────────────────────────────────────────────────┘
```

Criteria for Interruption

The test was interrupted for isolated or combined following
criteria.

TABLE II

```
EARLY EXERCISE TEST POST M.I.
        BEFORE DAY 20TH)

Criteria for interruption in 15 pts

Fatigue ..................... 11
Chest pain ................. 2
↘SBP ....................... 1
Target HR ................. 2
(90% of 220-age
VPB ......................... 4
```

Circulatory results and performance (TABLE III)

TABLE III

RESULTS OF EARLY EXERCISE TEST		
	REST	END OF EXERCISE
HR	80 ± 10	132 ± 16
SBP	126 ± 17	160 ± 23
DBP	82 ± 10	92 ± 12
Total work (Kpm)		4741 ± 4303*
*One patient performed : 19 940 Kpm Mean for the 14 others: 3 655 Kpm		

These results must be compared with those obtained in stable angina pectoris.

Maximal heart rate of hundred and thirty two is grossly equivalent to critical heart rate of patients with stable angina and triple vessel disease in our experience.

Indeed one patients, a high level cyclist performed a huge exercise at eighth day after anteroseptal infarction occuring as

he was climbing a pass in Pyrenees. The remaining fourteen
patients performed six hundred Kpm more than patients with stable
angina and triple vessel disease with the same symptom limited
heart rate.

The increase of blood pressure was normal. (TABLE IV)

TABLE IV

```
ECG CHANGES IN 15 PTS

(Beta-blockers .. 4 pts)
Nitrates .......15 pts)

Leads facing area of infarction :

- T < O ──────▶ T > O .................. 3
- T < O ──────▶ T "flat" ............... 2
- T < O ──────▶ T < O .................. 2
- S-T elevation (with T positivation)..... 6
- S-T depression ......................... 0
- No S-T or T changes .................... 2
  Other leads :
- S-T depression ......................... 7
- Mirror ................................. 3
- Primary ................................ 4
- No S-T changes ......................... 8
```

Some characteristic examples will be given.

1.   The first example is a "normal early exercise test after
     post M.I." (figure 1).

     The standard resting ECG displays a postero diaphragmatic
infarction with low lateral extension obvious in precordial leads
V5, V6.

     During exercise, there is slight S-T elevation in the posterior
lead ML5, mirror image in the septal lead, VE and increase in R
wave very often observed in the leads located to the border between
infarcted and non infarcted area.

     In this very sedentary man, the increase of heart rate and
blood pressure deserves no comment.

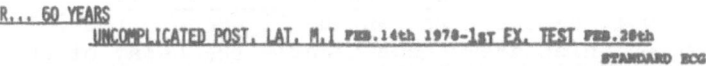

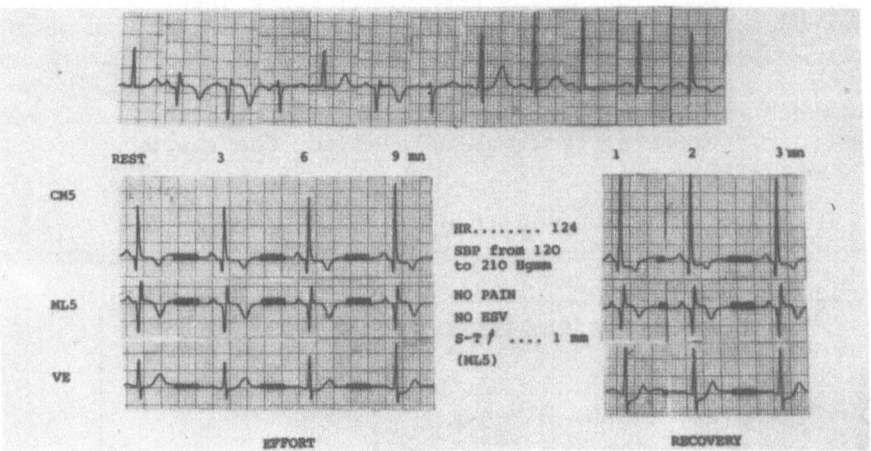

Figure 1.

But conversely it seems that absence of S-T elevation at early test is a good indicator of further functional and electrical improvement as illustrated on Figure 2, 13 days after onset there is a pattern of fresh anteroseptal infarction; during ET there was no further S-T elevation or T positivation in lead VE. Six months later, there is a considerable improvement both in ECG pattern with reduction of Q wave area and in functional capacity.

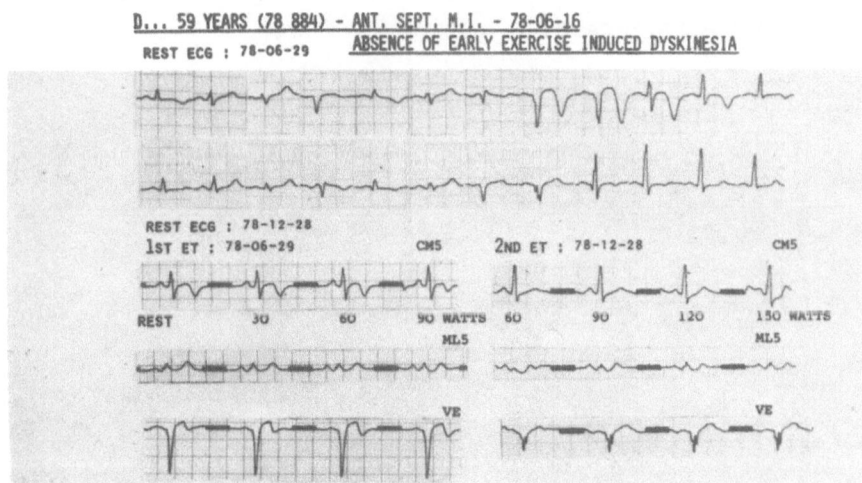

Figure 2.

Importance of drugs at the beginning of phase II. The safety
afforded by drugs is demonstrated on the figure 3: the S-T
segment depression, histogram shows clearly the delay of onset
of S-T segment depression during test immediately after sublingual
Nitroglycerin. This test leads to suppose a stenosis of LAD which
was confirmed by angiography.

"Delayed" early test after myocardial infarction. In 8
patients : early exercise test was delayed for the reasons
described on TABLE V.

TABLE V

```
"DELAYED" EARLY EXERCISE TEST (8PTS)

 - Patients exercised from day 20 th to day 50 th
   (mean day 30 th)

   Age : 50 ± 10 years (31 to 66)

 - Large anterior infarction with
   S-T elevation at rest ............... 5 cases

 - Angina ............................ 2 cases

 - Complicated acute phase ............ 1 case

   (diabetic coma and reversible renal failure)
```

F... 54 YEARS - (79 335) - PRINZMETAL ANGINA WITH S-T E IN V_1, V_2, V_3
70 % STENOSIS ON 2ND SEGMENT OF LAD
HYPERKINETIC CIRCULATORY PROFILE : ET WITH : NIFEDIPINE AND VERAPAMIL

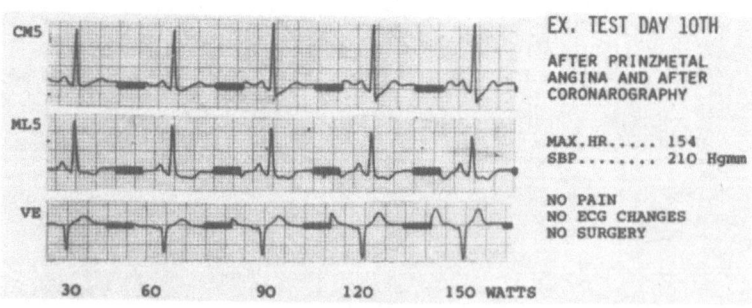

Figure 3.

Results of delayed exercise tests (TABLE VI). Most of these patients received several drugs and especially digitalis and diuretics were administrated in four.

The final results are slightly different of those of true early exercise tests. If the exercise capacity was grossly similar, the increase in heart rate, was higher, the increase in blood pressure lesser, these datas indicate a trend to left ventricular inadaptation to exercise.

TABLE VI

```
"DELAYED" EXERCISE TEST (8PTS)

Therapy:
  - Beta-blockers ................ 1 pts
  - Nitrates .................... 6 pts
  - Anti-arrythmic drugs ......... 4 pts
  - Digitalis and diuretics ...... 4 pts
               ----------
                  REST            END OF
                                  EXERCISE
  HR             82 ± 18         141 ± 31
  SBP           126 ± 19         157 ± 24
  DBP            84 ± 11          89 ± 17
  TOTAL WORK
    (Kpm)                       4083 ± 2561

  Criteria for cessation:
  - Fatigue : 4, Chest pain : 1
    Target HR : 1, Dyspnoea : 5
    Bouts of VPB : 1
```

Thus after infarction, besides further prospective studies on predictive value for long term prognosis, EET appears as a valuable tool in daily practice to separate patients into the following groups.

UNCOMPLICATED: Patients, who at the twentieth day may start with actual physical training.

COMPLICATED: by angina: following the predictible severity of ischemia from magnitude, duration, onset, location of S-T depression, it is possible to predict with good accuracy the severity of lesions and to perform angiogram in view of surgery.

- by large dyskinesia or aneurysm leading to meticulous exploration by multiscan echocardiography and ventriculography leading to resection by surgery.

- by arrythmias, commonly associated to previous complications, or isolated. A new exercise test will check the actual efficacy of anti-arrythmic drugs.

- by hypertension, hyperkinetic syndroms, all conditions needing beta-blockers of which the proper dose will be determined by comparative test.

Thus, besides further prospective studies of prediction value for long term prognosis. Early exercise test appears as a valuable clinical tool for proper management of patients.

II - EARLY EXERCISE TEST IN UNSTABLE ANGINA

Material and Methods

Unstable angina was defined by:

1.   Impending infarction with massive S-T changes still present between attacks of pain, without enzymes elevation or new Q wave.

2.   De novo angina with spontaneous attacks with or without effort angina.

3.   Prinzmetal variant.

In any case, a delay of five to seven days between the last attack of angina and the exercise test was respected. Drugs used in control of acute episode were not stopped for exercise test.

Conversely we did not take care of resting abnormalities of S-T and T waves.

- 25 patients exercised without any incident : ten were still under beta-blockers, all under high doses of long acting nitrates or Nifedipine.

The results are presented on Table VII.

This amount of work was similar to that performed by 70 patients with stable angina and one vessel disease studied in our institution. On the other hand the critical heart rate was lower (129 vs 142). This difference may be related with the administration of beta-blockers in ten patients.

TABLE VII

EARLY EXERCISE TEST DATA IN UNSTABLE ANGINA 25 male patients–Age:31 to 69–Mean:51		
	REST	EXERCISE
Heart rate	79 ± 16	129 ± 23
Syst. Blood P. (Hgmm)	136 ± 23	172 ± 24
Diast. Blood P. (Hgmm)	80 ± 16	91 ± 16
Total work (Kpm)	4832 ± 3580	

Interpretation of results in unstable angina. On this short group, we do not intend to offer statistical results. Moreover in absence of randomized study, the individual approach sustained by a careful follow up appears ethically correct.

Thus we divided our patients in the following groups:

TABLE VIII

INTERPRETATION OF EXERCISE TEST (ET) IN UNSTABLE ANGINA	No. of pts
- "Good ET" : NO coronarography : 10 patients	
- Asymptomatic (follow up one year)	8
- By passed 3 months after ET..............	1
- Myocardial infarction Death	1
	(68 years)
- "Normal ET" :	
- Prinzmetal variant (LAD stenosis 70%) ... (NIFEDIPINE)	1
- "Asymptomatic ET" with:	

- Resting S-T changes
    left ventricular thickening and
    normal coronary angiogram ....
	2

- "Poor ET" WITH coronarography : 12 patients by passed	7
- Inadequate run off	4
- Death during coronarography	1

- A good exercise test associated:

1.   An exercise capacity equal or superior to 120 watts for
     three minutes after three stages of three minutes duration
     at 30, 60, 90 watts.

2.   A S-T segment depression inferior to 3 mm in CM5 lead.

3.   An increase in systolic blood pressure at least of 4 hgcm

Ten patients belonged to this group: surgery was not proposed
whatever the results of coronary angiogram which was not performed
in some patients with excellent exercise test.

In this group, one patient had severe left anterior
descending artery stenosis and sustained 180 watts for three minutes
two weeks after attacks of resting angina and two years after
posterobasal infarction. The ET was interrupted for legs fatigue.
Surgery was cancelled. After three months he had dizziness
corresponding to bouts of ventricular tachycardia and was referred
to surgery.

Another patient, asymptomatic during exercise test died
suddenly after six months. He was 68 years old and the S-T
segment depression did not reach one mm.

One patient had Prinzmetal variant with left anterior
descending artery exhibiting a 70% stenosis. Exercise test was
performed after control of attacks by Nifedipine and coronarography
in order to decide between revascularisation or continuation of both
Nifedipine and Verapamil because of hyperkinetic circulation
(figure 3). The patient exercised to 150 watts for 3 minutes,
stopped for fatigue of legs without significant S-T changes. He
was left to medical therapy and remained asymptomatic for the
last ten months with normal activity as a general practitioner.

Two patients did not modify during exercise test important
resting S-T segment depression accompanying recurrent anginal
pains: coronary angiogram was normal but echocardiographic
examination revealed abnormal thickness of left ventricular wall
instead of absence of hypertension. Indeed, for a clinical point
of view, they belonged to the group of unstable angina.

Finally of 12 patients with poor exercise testing under or
without medical therapy, seven were by passed, four could not
because of poor run off and one died during coronarography.

Some practical difficulties in appraisal of exercise testing
results deserve some comments.

Drugs and exercise test interpretation. From the classical,
academic position ET should be done without any drug for proper
evaluation of the actual coronary status. Indeed in clinical
approach it appears more safe to start a first exercise test with
the patient under these drugs which allowed a five days period
free of any pain. If the result of first test are obviously bad,
it seems reasonable to look for feasibility of grafts by coronary
angiography. If the results appear satisfactory, we ask the
patient to interrupt beta-blockers, Nifedipine for 48 hours and
to start with a new exercise test.

On figure 4 is depicted a huge S-T segment depression at
60 watts (16.3 mm in CM5) which could be underestimated by
nitrates 16 days before (78-09-10) when the patient came as an
out patient for evaluation of some attacks of spontaneous angina.
After the second test surgery was rapidly performed and a post-
operative test (79-01-31) show the disappearance of S-T segment
depression.

Figure 5 shows how the suppression of drugs in a young
patient with double vessel disease reduced the exercise capacity
from 150 to 90 watts leading to surgery in spite of asymptomatic
status with medical therapy. After two grafts, there was no
longer pain, even with cessation of drugs, at 180 watts.

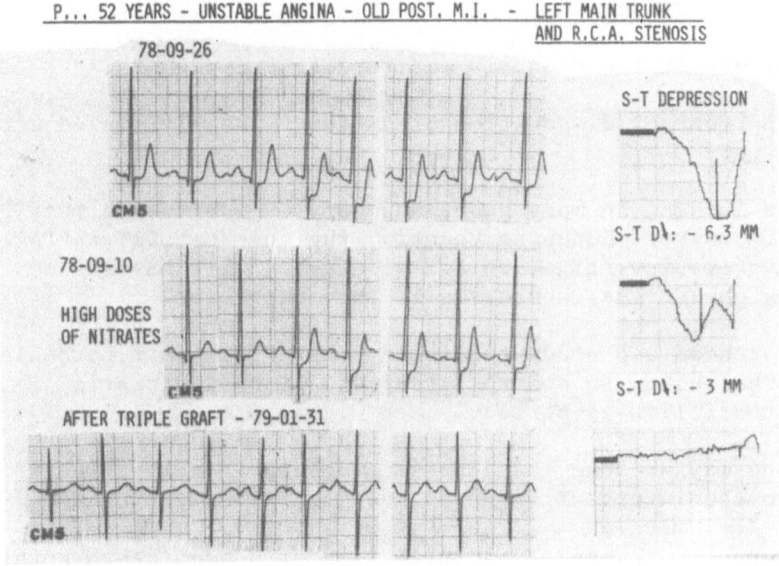

Figure 4.

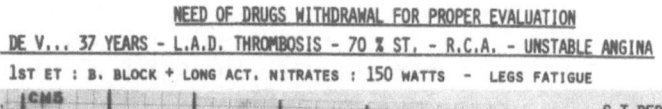

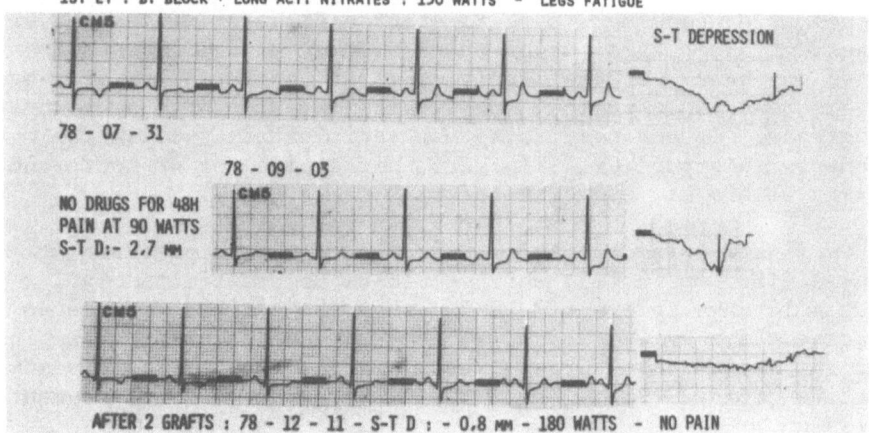

Figure 5.

DISCUSSION

Commonly accepted strategy in management of unstable angina is:

1. Control of chest pain by vigorous therapy

2. Coronarography

3. Surgery if the stenosis and run off are proper

4. Then further disparition of angina is hastly linked with
    surgery.

This is inexact in many cases and very expensive; we must be
aware that in most of European Country, the cost/benefit ratio
of every invasive investigation and of surgery will have to be
revisited by physicians themselves in the next years.

In any randomized study published, there is a fair percentage
of patients belonging to control group who are asymptomatic
throughout the follow up period.

Thus one may presume that the same percentage of patients
belonging to the intervention group has been wrongly operated.

Moreover, in prevention of infarction or sudden death nothing
has not yet definitely proven: there is no difference in
mortality or incidence of new myocardial infarction. But the pain
is more often relieved in operated groups.

Then a different strategy relying on early exercise test appears useful in unstable angina and may be proposed according to Table IX.

TABLE IX

PERIODIC COMPARATIVE

EXERCISE TEST

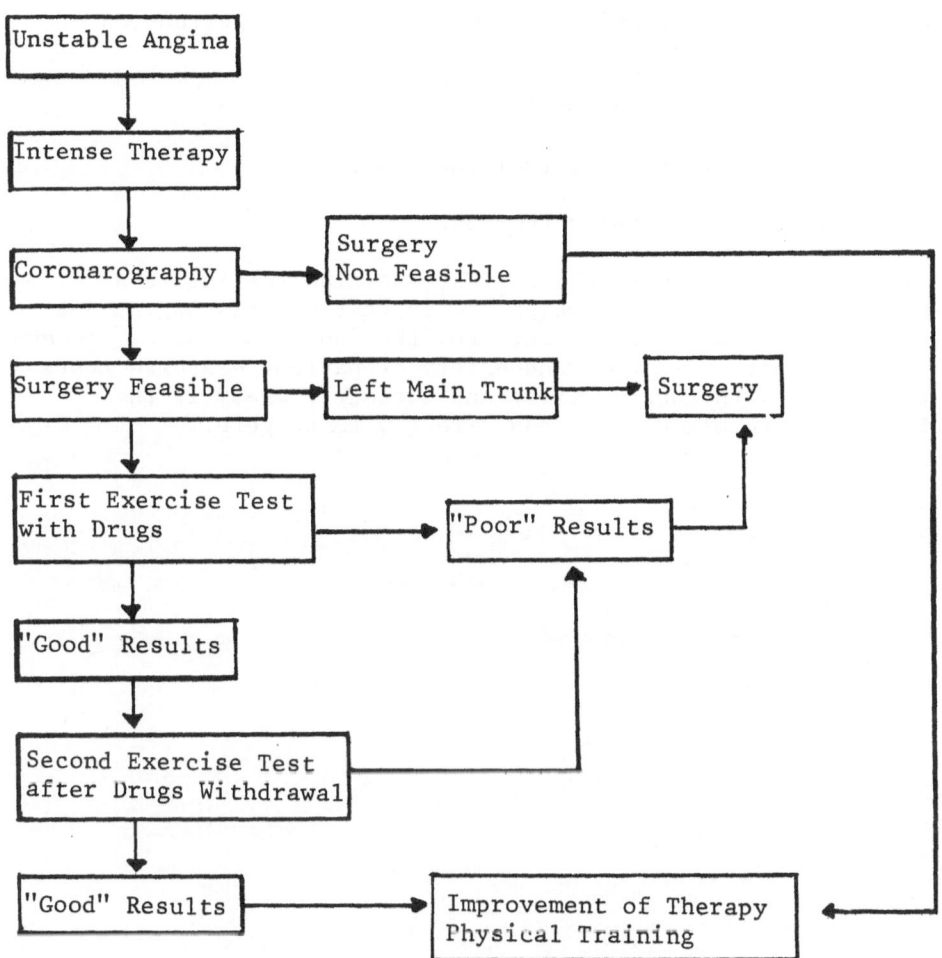

This policy in our experience avoided too many patients for several years, a hasty surgery submitted to the automatic schema: unstable angina = coronary stenosis = surgery.

CONCLUSION

After myocardial infarction, early exercise test brings help to:

1. Identification of latent complications such as cardiac failure, dyskinesia, arrythmia, angina, hypertension or hypotension during exercise.

2. Reinsurance of the patient

3. Planning of physical training sessions

4. Adjustment of proper therapy.

After controlled unstable angina, exercise testing is a safety rail which allows to weigh the indications of surgery not from a pre-established policy but from the individual data. Indeed to combine proper evaluation and safety of patient exercise tests should be done with therapy first and without therapy if the results of first test do not lead directly to surgery.

SYMPTOM LIMITED EXERCISE TEST IN APPRAISAL OF ANTI-ANGINAL DRUGS

J. P. Broustet, J. F. Cherrier, P. Martin Neuville, and
P. Guern

Département des Epreuves d'Effort
Hopital Cardiologique du Haut Leveque
33604 - Pessac, France

INTRODUCTION

Critical Review of Traditional Trials.

These trials relied on drug administration for several weeks
or months. The patients were asked to keep a diary of anginal attacks and the number of Nitroglycerin pills (NTG) used. These
trials used commonly a placebo period and a drug period with the
help of a cross over.

Pitfalls of traditional trials. They do not take into account
the clinical evolution of the so called "stable angina pectoris" its
evolution is largely variable throughout the time from one patient
to another and within rather short periods.

Moreover the increase of anginal attacks with placebo leads
the patient to limit its activity. The result may be a paradoxal
decrease of anginal attacks and of NTG consumption!

Conversely if an active drug is given, the patient will have
more activity and will get more frequent episodes : as he will
not be clearly aware of the increase in the level of triggering
exercise or as he will not properly quote them in his diary the
physician will just note that the drug increased the number of
attacks and the NTG consumption!

Moreover the temperature may change : if the placebo period
fits with a warm period the crisis will spontaneously decrease.
On the other hand if the drug period occurs during cold season or
during an overdose of professional activity this will lead to an
increase of angina.

49

Contamination by other drugs is not rare during long duration
trials. Many physicians and even cardiologists do not willingly
accept that their patient remain with numerous attacks. Thus
if the placebo period is followed by aggravation or if the tested
drug is unefficient the patient is to be pulled out of the trial
for he received classical and efficient therapy.

At least in latin countries this way is very frequent and
quite impossible to avoid if the duration trial is superior to
one month.

Placebo is not without risk.

During effort, angina, a number of patients do have bouts of
extrasystoles which may be dangerous.

Moreover if one wants to get a significant reduction of
the number of anginal attacks one must deal with patients who do
have many daily episodes of pain that is now rare in stable angina.
Indeed the very sedentary life of most of the patients is per se
a limiting factor of anginal pain even if their exercise capacity
if very poor.

Thus the only patients who may enter in long term trials are
usually extremely limited, have a triple vessel disease of which
the course may be very short. It is well known how poor is the
prognosis of a patient suffering angina while walking on the
level, bathing, driving.

For these reasons administration of a placebo for several
weeks is often discouraging for the patient who thinks he is
using a drug. His family doctor may consider this situation as
unacceptable.

Thus, it has been considered that the assessment of antianginal drugs by means of careful exercise test was a better way
to use.

Value of Drug Assessment by Means of Symptom Limited Exercise
Testing (SLET)

Possibility to attend the anginal attack SLET makes it possible
to put the patients in the proper conditions which will allow both
a pragmatic and explaining study of the activity of the tested drug.

Collected informations concerning circulatory and electrocardiographic data and their changes with the drug will be very
valuable when compared to control data.

Safety and litigation problems. Provided a careful selection

of patients which rejects patients with too low anginal threshold or
with malignant arrythmias occuring at the time of pain, drug-assess-
ment by means of SLET appear to be safe. We have been testing drugs
in more than 250 patients with effort angina; among those who had
coronary angiogram the mean number of stenosed vessels was 2.7.

The repetition of tests in different conditions correspond
to more than 1500 SLET without any serious complications.

Co-operation of the patient has therapeutic side effects.
As emphasized by Blackburn: exercise test creates a link between
patient and cardiologist. When actively involved in drug trial,
the patient has the feeling to participate by himself to his own
management and if the tested drugs are effective he will get a
favourable feeling of hope.

Studies on combinations of drugs. SLET not only allow us to
compare a drug with a placebo or a reference drug (such as NTG),
but also to study the combination of several drugs and their
potentiation. NTG and beta-blockers, beta-blockers and calcium
blockers for example.

Determination of duration of activity of a simple dose by
asking the patient to repeart the SLET for example 1H, 3H, 5H, 12H,
24H after drug administration, it is possible to determine the
adequate posology of drugs.

Finally these facilities do have practical implications
beyond a scientific trial. Even when the patient does not belong
to a selected group, it remains easy by means of comparative
exercise test with single, double dose, combination of drugs,
to select the best combination and the proper posology for daily
life.

Indeed the follow up has proven that best SLET make the best
daily life in stable angina pectoris.

METHODOLOGY

Protocole of Symptom Limited Exercise Tests

Ergometer. At least in France cycloergometer is usually
employed. It must be accurately calibrated, electrically
braked. It allows a proper control of arterial pressure.

The increment in carefully standardized: whatever the tested
drug, we use a progression of 30 watts every three minutes: the
first stage starts at 30 watts. This allows some comparison with
previous trials.

<u>Criteria for cessation</u>. Angina is the most important end point in anti-anginal drugs assessment as this kind of drug is supposed to prevent or suppress anginal attacks! Thus any patient selected for trials must have not only exercise induced ischemia but also exercise induced angina during the control test.

With drugs, pain should be the criteria for cessation. But if the drug is effective pain will no longer appear and will be replaced by fatigue of legs, or dyspnoea or arrythmias.

Whatever its amplitude isolated S-T segment depression is never a criteria for interruption.

Display of electrocardiogram must be permanent, with standard twelve leads before and after exercise. During exercise it is necessary to use leads very sensitive for ischemia so that ischemia can be better quantified. For this purpose we use routinely the CM5 lead which provides the most important amplitude of S-T segment depression regarding the amplitude of R wave.

Moreover we have been using for the last two years the "CASE" system from Marquette which provides a quantification of ischemia displayed by means of histograms of S-T depression and S-T slope throughout the time. This device is very useful for statistical purposes.

Parameters Studied

They are not sophisticated:

resting heart rate

critical or symptom limited or maximal heart rate

heart rate for the same stage of exercise

work load for the same value of heart rate

resting blood pressure

maximal or symptom limited blood pressure

double product: heart rate x systolic blood pressure at rest and at submaximal or maximal work load

total work performed

S-T segment depression: at same subcritical heart rate and work load and at the time of cessation of exercise.

The patient being his own control, the paired-t-tests will allow to compare these different parameters in short groups of 15 to 25 patients.

A variance analyses will check the presence or the absence of influence of repetition of tests provided a random allocation between placebo or drug has been used for every patient.

Selection of patients is the most difficult part of this procedure: from a clinical point of view one must deal exclusively with stable patients describing a reproducible exercise angina in daily life, without pattern of anterior infarction which makes impossible analysis of CM5 lead. A careful clinical examination coupled with bidimensional echocardiography is necessary to reject those patients having cardiac enlargement, cardiac failure, global hypokinesia of left ventricule, valvular disease such as aortic stenosis.

Moreover one must check the patients willing to participate actively to the trial and to accept exercise induced chest pain as a criteria for cessation of repeated exercise tests.

At least one must reject patients with limiting factors capable to appear during exercise if the assayed drug decreases angina: thus a patient with legs arteritis may have angina after seven minutes of exercise and after improvement by drug, he will exhibit intermittent claudication at the 8th minute! The same is true for respiratory insufficiency.

Nobody will be admitted to trials before preliminary symptom limited exercise test which will allow to check his aptitude and the proper S-T segment depression; the absence of severe arrythmias at onset of ischemia.

The patients to be selected should have:

a normal resting S-T segment in CM5

a progressive S-T depression during exercise

a chest pain compelling to cessation of test,this pain is quoted in four classes in our laboratory:

Class 1:   retrosternal feeling of heat or weight without definite pain

Class 2:   mild but tolerable pain

Class 3:   disagreeable retrosternal pain leading to cessation of test

Class 4:   acute frank retrosternal pain leading to immediate
           uptake of Nitroglycery. Indeed this last eventuality
           is uncommon

These criteria for selection constitute a guarantee of
homogeneity of different sets of different patients studied at
different periods. This allows us to know if such or such drug
is frankly different to others or not. Moreover any trial with
any new drug is coupled to a comparison with the answer to sublingual nitroglycerin which thus remains a common factor throughout
the different trials.

One must avoid to select patients with too low anginal
threshold for they may have left main true stenosis or severe
cardiac failure. Conversely if the pain appears after the 150 watts
stage the physological limits are very near and the capacity of
production is limited by legs fatigue.

Phenomenon of training. Some very complicated protocols
require six to eight successive exercise tests within three or
four days. Thus familiarization with pain, and training effect
may induce a bias. But duration and level of SLET are actually
very short to provide training effect. Any way a variance
analysis is sometimes useful to check that there was not
"sequential effect".

Protocols

They will be adjusted both to the target and to realistic clinical possibilities.

Pharmacological aims. At time of protocole planning, the maker
and the expert do define carefully the purpose of trial: if
one search for appraisal of antianginal effect the schedule depend
on kinetics of the drug. Sometimes determination of duration of
action is to be made; for example: one will compare the effects
of sublingual TNT to those of a so called long acting nitrate or
beta-blocker taken one hour, three hours, six, seventy four
hours before another SLET.

Sometimes one looks for the proper dosage: the same patients
will perform every day or two days an SLET, with single, double,
triple dose and placebo allocated in random order varying with
each patient.

Clinical constraints. It is obvious that anginal patients
are not robots. One must take into account their disponibility,
willingness motivation and hospital constraints.

Usually patients are referred for coronary angiogram which
is delayed until achievement of drug trial.

In our institution we developed for ten years a training department for patients with stable angina not willing or not able for technical contra-indication to have coronary by pass. They form a nucleus trained to exercise test and exercise induced chest pain and quite suitable for purpose of trial. In absence of drugs serial SLET are perfectly reproducible.

RESULTS

It is not possible to summarize all the protocoles we used for the last five years. Let us recall some of them.

Trial of Sublingual Nitroglycerin (SLNTG)

SLNTG remains our reference drug or control drug used as a complementary control in other trial dealing with other drugs.

In some patients trial of single and double dose of beta-blockers were carried out. The main data are:

1. Circulatory changes (heart rate; blood pressure) are poorly changed with double dose.

2. There was no relationship between the blood concentration of drug from one patient to another but in every patient a good correlation between dose and blood concentration.

3. The mean value of exercise capacity was poorly increased by double dose, but when looking at individual results, there was very different features.

Double dose induced exercise cardiac failure in some patients, leading to a decrease of exercise capacity because of severe dyspnoea even when pain no longer appeared.

In other patients with normal left ventricular function and high critical heart rate the double dose provided significant improvement.

Protocole. After a first control SLET, and a recovery period of 3 minutes duration SLNTG dose (0.75 mg (NATIROSE)) is given. One minute later a new SLET starts.

In these conditions in a group of 46 patients, we found an increase of 46% in exercise capacity, a decrease of critical S-T segment depression of 14% in spite of an increase in critical heart rate from a mean value of 122 beats/minute to 138 beats/minute (figure 1). At the same subcritical heart rate the reduction of S-T segment depression was of 57%.

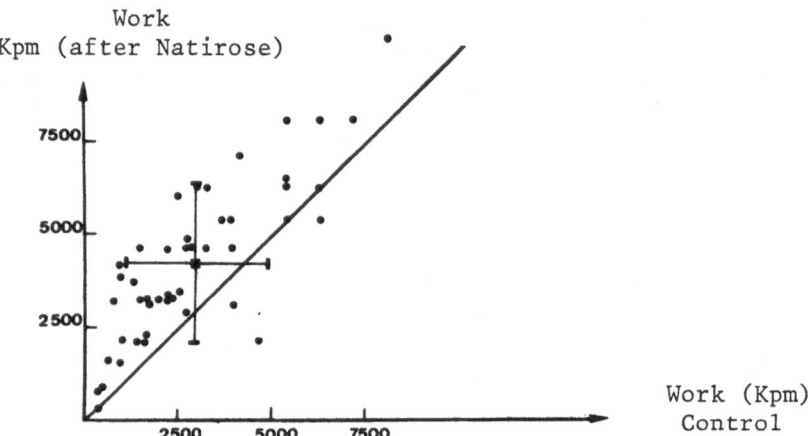

Fig. 1. Progression of effort capacity under Trinitrine preventative.
         Control: 2900±2000 Kpm
         Natirose: 4250±2145 Kpm

Before SLNTG all patients stopped for angina. After SLNTG
pain occurred only in 65% of cases giving place to legs fatigue
or dyspnoea.

The placebo effect of SLNTG was tested. One day patient
received SL placebo SLNTG, the other day LSNTG, the order of
administration was randomized. The progression of exercise
capacity by regard to control value was 12% with placebo 54%
with SLNTG.

Beta-Blockers. Whatever the drug assayed (Pindolol,Penbutolol
Propranolol, Practolol, Metoprolol, Atenolol) with doses
equivalent to 80 or 120 mg of Propranolol/24 hr, the increase of
exercise capacity ranged from 42 to 64%. When we added SLNTG
to beta-blockers the results were always better with than with
SLNTG or Beta-blockers alone. When comparing SLNTG done to
beta-blockers alone the better results always favoured SLNTG.

The schedule was:

Long acting nitrates (LAN). Daily practice provides
convincing data for a short duration of effects of so called
long acting nitrates. Three times/a day routine prescription
appeared not safe. To check this hypothesis we administered a
capsule of LAN or placebo to four patients. Every patient
received four 40 days, either placebo in randomized order
different for each patient. Three hours later he performed a
SLET. Thus there were 80 LSET with LAN and 80 with placebo.

In the conditions, we could not find any significant
difference concerning exercise capacity, critical heart rate,
blood pressure, S-T segment depression values.

Nitroglycerin ointment. 30 anginal patients received
either 15 mg (in 15) either 30 mg (in 15) of nitroglycerin
ointment or placebo in randomized allocation. They performed an
exercise test 30 and 180 minutes after ointment or NTG or placebo.
Moreover they were with control test and sublingual NTG. In these
conditions, the critical heart rate (HR) and the total work
(Kpm) were:

	HR	Kpm (15 mg)	Kpm (30 mg)
For control test	118		
After SL NTG	137	5417	3600
After placebo			
after 15 minutes	129	3844	3419
after 180 minutes	121	3703	2931
After NTG ointment			
control test	118		
after 15 minutes	129	5540	4411
after 180 minutes	130	4670	4493

There was significant difference after three hours and a double
dose was more effective at the end of three hours.

Calcium blockers. We studied Nifedipine by the means of
following/protocole.

We used a single dose of 20 mg given by sublingual administration.

Day one: control test: 8h30
          SLNTG test just after control test

Day two: 8h AM: administration of 20 mg of Nifedipine or
                  placebo
          8h30:   1st exercise test
          11h: 2nd exercise test

Day three: idem with placebo or Nifedipine

Three hours after aministration Nifedipine provided the
same improvement as SLNTG in terms of: exercise capacity,
increase in critical heart rate, decrease in S-T segment
depression. This was quite different to data observed after the
so called long acting nitrates.

CRITICAL APPRAISAL OF THESE SHORT TERM TRIALS

Long term activity was not checked. Such an approach does not
allow to make sure of long term effect, but by performing
comparative SLET after 6 months with drug and after withdrawal
it is possible to provide a proper answer.

Tolerance and side effects. They cannot be appraised and
long duration administration remains mandatory for this purpose.
But one may lighten the burden of cardiologists by avoiding them
to deal both with efficiency and tolerance. They just have to
look for tolerance provided that repeated SLET will check the long
term effect. Thus, they may devote strictly to tolerance evaluation
which is far more simple and accurate.

CONCLUSION

Assessment of antianginal drugs by means of repeated SLET is
certainly the simplest and most accurate way. Indeed this procedure
does not dispense from hemodynamic studies providing a better
comprehension of mechanism of action.

These trial lead to say that up to now the best therapy of
exercise induced angina is the combination of little dosages of
beta-blockers and calcium inhibitor provided that the patient
had neither byadycardia, neither hypotension non cardiac failure.

In the same perspective assessment of results of revascularization is very objective and simple and allow an accurate judgement
sometimes less enthusiastic than it appears in many surgical
papers.

RATIONALE OF PHYSICAL TRAINING IN PATIENTS WITH ANGINA PECTORIS

J. J. Kellermann, Ch. Lapidot, E. Ben-Ari,
M. Hayet, and Y. Drory

Cardiac Evaluation and Rehabilitation Institute
Chaim Sheba Medical Center
Tel Hashomer and Tel Aviv University Medical School
Israel

Some 18 years ago, as we started on our first steps in rehabilitating the post myocardial infarction patients, we soon found out that the main problem we are facing is the patient with angina pectoris (1). In a preliminary study involving 93 patients after myocardial infarction with a mean age of 52 years without angina pectoris, we obtained a physical work capacity of about 80% of the norm as established at our laboratory (according to healthy individuals matched by age and sex).

This relatively high PWC was obtained without rehabilitation and before the patient returned to full activity (2).

In 102 patients with angina pectoris in the same age group, a mean PWC of 54% was found. It is obvious that the latter group was significantly incapacited and almost all of them belonged to class late II and early III of the New York Heart Association Functional Classification. While the post myocardial infarction patients without angina pectoris reached an exercise testing target heart rate of 151 $\pm$ 3,8 beats/min. (b/m) the angina pectoris group could not continue after target heart rates of 125 $\pm$ 6,5 b/m.

Lactic acid was examined in the arterialized capillary blood. While the PWC (assessed by a multistage near maximal testing protocol) at target heart rates of 150 b/m in healthy and in asymptomatic coronary patients showed a lactic acid concentration of 45,7 $\pm$ 11,3 mg% and in coronary patients 45,2 $\pm$ 6,9 mg%, in the angina pectoris group at target heart rates 125 b/m we found 24,5 $\pm$ 3,9 mg%. (3)

These findings clearly indicate that, while applying a
rehabilitation program based also on physical training, our
main concern should be concentrated on the patient with angina
pectoris. In preparing a physical training program for these
patients, one must consider that a coronary patient without a
significant impairment of the pliability of his coronary arteries,
will have the same response mechanism as a healthy individual,
i.e. he will meet the increased myocardial oxygen demand during
physical exertion by a consequent rise in coronary flow and
probably also a more economic extraction of oxygen in the coronary
capillary region (4,5).

One of the most striking and early findings in our studies
was the fact that, when heart rate, oxygen consumption, oxygen
pulse and double product in various work loads obtained in
healthy individuals are compared to those in patients with coronary
heart disease, no significant differences in the aforementioned
parameters are found. Of course, this linearity can be seen only
up to the individual exercise level in which relative steady
state conditions are maintained and it is dependent on the
functional capacity of each examinee (3).

These findings make it possible to prepare individually
adjusted training programs for the coronary patient with a maximal
margin of safety. On the other hand, the intensity of our programs
applied during the first years of our activity, proved to be
moderately effective and sometimes even ineffective in reaching
any physiological results in the angina pectoris patient. While
the same kind of program applied in the asymptomatic patient
resulted always in a beneficial physiological effect.

Myocardial oxygen demand increases by physical training and
it is known that in the angina pectoris patient there is an
impaired relation between myocardial oxygen consumption and total
body VO_2 during exercise. The therapeutic modality of physical
training in patients with angina pectoris is based on the
assumption that effective training could eventually reduce the
discrepancy between oxygen demand and supply, the goal of therapy
being, that the increased demand will eventually cause an increased
supply. While in healthy individuals such an increase can be
achieved by rise in coronary flow, as mentioned earlier, this rise
can be reached by decreasing the resistance of the coronary
vessels. As we have said, this will be possible only in the healthy
individual and in the patient without significant obstruction of
his coronary vessels or without significant impairment of the
pliability and still capable of dilating resistance of the
coronary vessels. (4, 5, 6).

The problem starts with an increased demand of the coronary
flow in patients with coronary heart disease, who have highly
obstructive disease and will therefore have difficulties in
increasing oxygen supply. Inadequate flow distribution will cause
a subsequent decrease in myocardial contractility and result in
the impairment of myocardial performance (4).

Our unsatisfactóry findings in the first years of our work,
led to the development of high intensity training programs based
on the individual angina pectoris threshold heart rate (7,8).
A 4 months training program on mechanically braked bicycles and
based on intensities of 55% and 90% of the individual angina
pectoris threshold heart rate, proved to give a sufficient
response as to the capabilities of the patient to adapt himself
to regular physical training. If an effective cardio-respiratory
response to training in the angina pectoris patients is reached
within 16 weeks, we continue with the conservative measures and
o ur comprehensive rehabilitation program. If there is no sufficient
training effect within this time period, the patient is transferred
to cine-angiography an d in 85% of these patients subsequent
coronary artery surgery was performed.

THE PHYSIOLOGICAL EFFECT OF TRAINING

The hemodynamic background and various physiological aspects
of physical training in coronary patients have been studied
extensively during the past decade. As it has been stated by us
earlier there is a similar central and peripheral circulatory
response to training in healthy individuals as compared to
coronary patients. Naturally this is only the case for patients
who are capable to undergo a physical training program.and
fulfill the clinical requirements for acceptance to such a program.
Naturally the training intensity will differ in patients after
myocardial infarction who do or do not suffer from angina pectoris.
It is well accepted that physical training decreases the heart
rate and the myocardial oxygen demand at a given work task. The
systolic blood pressure for a given load decreases while an
augmented stroke volume is found, especially in low to moderate
work loads. The arteriovenus oxygen difference remains unchanged
at submaximal work levels but increases at maximal work. Muscle
blood flow is decreased during submaximal work and increased
during maximal work. Oxygen extraction in the working muscle
improves. The muscular oxygen potential is improved after
training indicated by a larger mitochondrial mass and increased
concentration of oxydative enzymes. In patients with angina pectoris
we foun d within a 4 months training program a significant decrease
of heart rate, systolic blood pressure, double product (HR x SBP),
oxygen pulse and triple product (SBP x HR x LVET) for a given
work task (see figures 1-5 and Table 1 and 2).

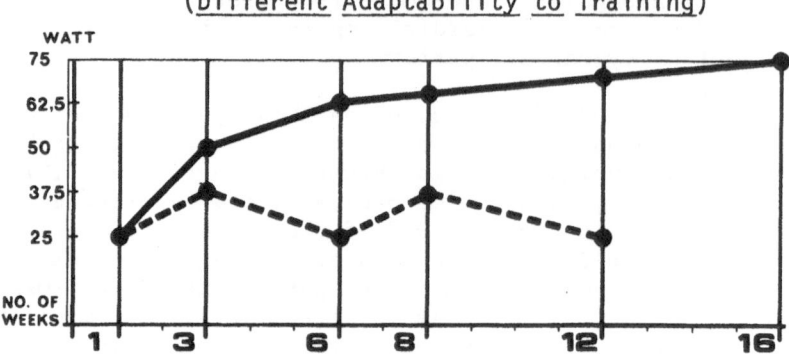

Fig. 1. Different adaptability to prolonged physical training in
         patients with angina pectoris. The group of patients
         incapable of reaching a training effect within 12 weeks
         are transferred to cine-angiography of the coronary
         arteries.

         (Reproduced with permission of S. Karger AG, Basel New
         York from Kellermann J.J., Denolin H. (eds.) Critical
         Evaluation of Cardiac Rehabilitation. P.35, 1977).

Different Training Intensities

        In order to assess the importance of the training intensity
and a possible placebo effect we have studied the effect of
different training programs in 33 patients after myocardial
infarction with angina pectoris (9). 15 of these 33 patients
underwent a low intensity program based on calisthenics while
the remaining 18 patients were switched after 40 weeks of
calisthenics training to an high intensity ergometric training.
The patients were divided according to the severity of pain
during stress testing and daily activities, into two groups:
(1) those with severe pain started intensive (90% of pain
threshold heart rate), prolonged (continuous 30 min.) ergometric
training and patients with lesser complaints who continued with
the calisthenics program. The results of the latter group,
after 18 months of training, did not reveal a significant change
in submaximal heart rate (HR), systolic blood pressure (SBP),
O_2 pulse, double or triple product (DP, TP). However, in 20% of
the patients a higher pain threshold HR was tolerated and the

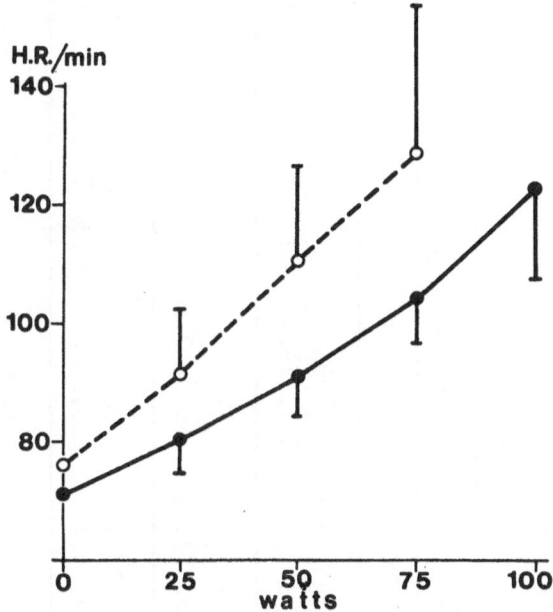

Fig. 2.   Shows the heart rate before (---) and after (——) a
          four months training program.

higher DP reached before onset of anginal pain. Ergometric
training caused a significant change in all the circulatory
parameters mentioned above. In addition, four patients
increased their pain threshold of both HR and DP. 20% of the
patients increased their maximal HR and DP, regardless of
exercise intensity. The lowering of the systolic blood pressure
x heart rate product (DP) and the decrease of the triple product
(DP x LVET) is related to appearance of bradycardia and a decrease
in systemic arterial pressure, the latter findings seems to be an
important factor when evaluating the mechanical work of the
heart after training.

TABLE 1

CIRCULATORY MEASUREMENTS IN PATIENTS WITH ANGINA PECTORIS
BEFORE AND AFTER
4 MONTH INTENSIVE ERGOMETRIC TRAINING PROGRAMS

LOAD AND TIME	HR (Beats/min) BEFORE	AFTER	P	Blood pressure (mmHg) BEFORE	AFTER	P	SBP x HR BEFORE	AFTER	P
REST	83 ± 11.3	78 ± 8.08	NS	135/90 ± 17.5/9.9	135/90 ± 17.5/9.9	NS	12057 ± 2655	10549 ± 1296	NS
5 min at 55 per cent of pain threshold heart rate	109 ± 4.0	92 ± 4.0	<0.01	155/88 ± 17.8/8.0	136/87 ± 15.0/10.0	NS	14134 ± 1647	12191 ± 1796	<0.05
10 min at 90 per cent of pain threshold heart rate	121 ± 8.2	109 ± 8.8	<0.01	167/84 ± 19.4/8.7	138/87 ± 13.7/8.3	<0.05	20364 ± 3018	17501 ± 2100	<0.01
25 min at 90 per cent of pain threshold heart rate	123 ± 14.5	113 ± 8.1	<0.05	164/87 ± 18.3/8.8	164/89 ± 17.3/8.6	NS	20916 ± 3610	18419 ± 2333	<0.01

NS: not significant

TABLE 2

OXYGEN CONSUMPTION (VO$_2$) AND O$_2$ PULSE IN PATIENTS WITH ANGINA PECTORIS BEFORE AND AFTER 4-MONTH INTENSIVE ERGOMETRIC TRAINING PROGRAMME

LOAD AND TIME	O$_2$ PULSE (ML O$_2$/BEAT)			VO$_2$L/MIN		
	BEFORE	AFTER	P	BEFORE	AFTER	P
REST	4.2 ± 1.4	4.4 ± 1.04	NS	0.343 ±0.020	0.342 ±0.025	NS
5 min at 55 per cent of pain threshold heart rate	7.7 ± 1.8	8.7 ± 1.5	<0.05	0.764 ±0.058	0.764 ±0.065	NS
10 min at 90 per cent of pain threshold heart rate	9.8 ± 1.5	9.9 ± 1.8	NS	1.230 ±0.101	1.038 ±0.095	<0.05
25 min at 90 per cent of pain threshold heart rate	8.9 ± 1.7	9.8 ± 2.0	<0.05	1.119 ±0.100	1.100 ±0.090	NS

NS: not significant

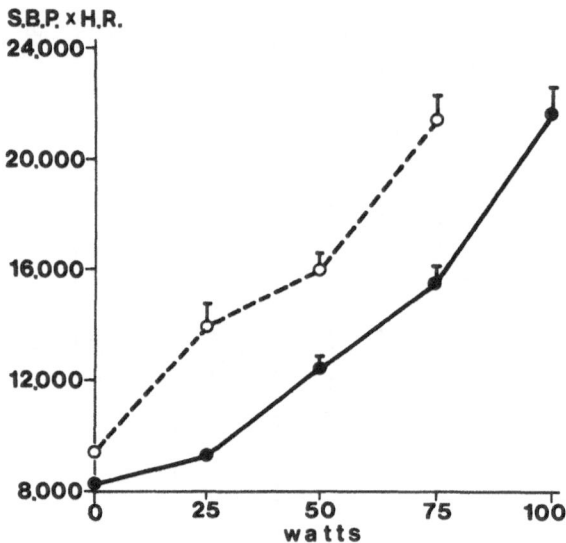

Fig. 3.   Shows the double products (SBP x HR) before (---) and
          after (---) a four months program. Can be seen that there
          is a significant decrease of the DP in each work load.
          After 4 months higher angina pectoris threshold DP's are
          obtained.

Cardiocirculatory Effect of Prolonged Training

In a further study Ben-Ari et al (10) have examined at our
laboratory the effect of prolonged intensive training on cardio-
respiratory response in angina pectoris patients. The prolonged
work was investigated in 15 patients after transmural myocardial
infarction. The patients suffered from angina pectoris of different
severity. Based on an individually determined pain threshold heart
rate the following two relative work loads were obtained; 55 per
cent and 90 per cent of threshold heart rate. Training was
monitored using the 10-channel Siemens radio-telemetry system,
and consisted of 30 minutes continuous pedalling, twice per week.
Pretraining results showed a substantial increase in heart rate
(HR 12 ± 8,2) and systolic blood pressure (SBP 15 mmHg) between
the 5th and the 10th minute of work and decrease in O_2 consumption
(VO_2 1/min) and O_2 pulse between the 15th and 30th minute of
exercise. Training resulted in the following changes: Decreased
heart rate at rest and during work (p ⩽ 0.01). Systolic blood
pressure did not rise up to the 15th minute of work. Oxygen
consumption increased gradually, reaching a steady state after 15

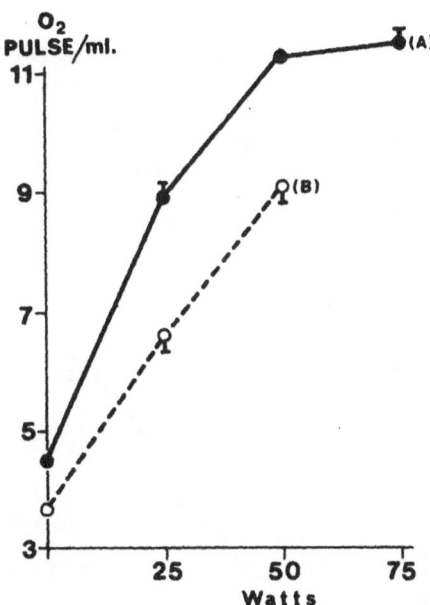

Fig. 4. The oxygen pulse before (A) and after (B) a four months
program. A significant increase in O_2 pulse can be seen
indicating an increase in stroke volume after training.

minutes of work. O_2 pulse increased gradually and remained
constant during the last 15 minutes of work. SBP x HR product
decreased significantly ($p \leqslant 0.05 - 0.01$) at rest and during work.
Clinically there was a pronounced decrease in severity and
frequency of angina pectoris along with increased work time before
onset of pain. The data show that intensive prolonged training
may result in improvement of the physiological adaptive mechanism
of patients with angina pectoris to continuous physical stress.

The ability to perform continuous exercise depends on adequate
supply of oxygenated blood and fuel for combustion for the working
muscles. Data on favourable effect of training on myocardial
infarction have not been consistant. Some investigators (11)
most of whom used moderate exercise routines reported unimproved
left ventricular function. We should like to mention that in our
study intensive training resulted in significant lower systolic
blood pressure from the start up to 15th minute of exercise,
suggesting a reduction in total vascular resistance and
contractile work of the left ventricle during this time.

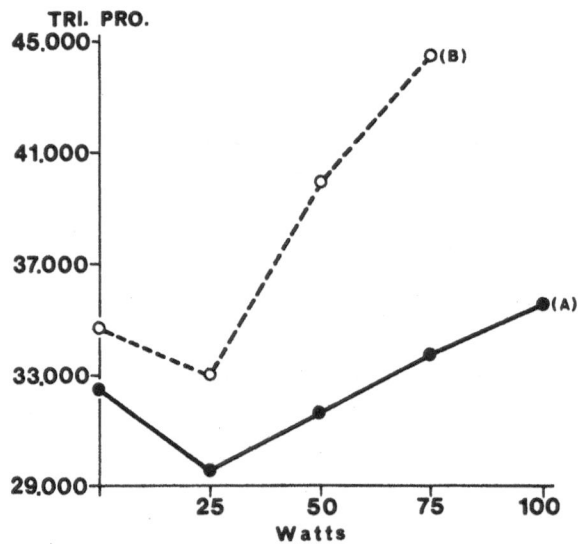

Fig. 5.   The triple product (HR b/m x SBP mmHg x LVET (sec)) before
          (B) and after (A) a 4 months training program. A marked
          decrease of the triple product has been found for each
          given work task after training.

OXYGEN PULSE

At our laboratory the oxygen pulse (oxygen consumption
ml x heart rate) has been extensively studied during the last ten
years. We should like to report in short about some investigations
concerning especially the angina pectoris patients. The oxygen
pulse is being considered a relative measure of stroke volume (12).
In a 4 months training program we have found a significant increase
of the oxygen pulse for a given work task in patients with angina
pectoris. (fig.4).   In the group of patients without
cardiocirculatory adaptation to training the observation was
made that during increasing exercise induced pain, the oxygen
pulse decreases and the double product increases. The decrease
in the oxygen pulse would indicate a decrease in stroke volume
as a result of hypoxia, while the enhanced double product
indicates an increased myocardial oxygen demand. When nitroglycerin
was administered sublingually during pain, the oxygen pulse
immediately increased and the double product decreased. The
patient could then continue his exercise session. In patients
experiencing a mild, not increasing pain during exercise
performance, which disappeared during continuation, the oxygen
pulse did not decrease – despite a significant increase of the
double product. The patients with a "walk through" phenomenon had
an increased double product threshold at the end of exercise
performance. The oxygen pulse constitutes in our opinion, one
of the most important hemodynamic parameters in the assessment of
the effect of physical training in patients with angina pectoris.
In about 20–25% of our patients with angina pectoris, the angina
pectoris threshold heart rate (ATHR) increased as a consequence
of training.

ATHR as a Prognostic Sign

A comparative study prepared at our laboratory by Hayet et al,
(13) showed that in a 5 years follow up, the mortality in angina
pectoris patients with ATHR of less than 120 b/m was 25.3% in an
untrained control group, as against 9,3% in trained intervention
group. In the group of patients with ATHR above 120 b/m, there
was again a significant difference in the 5 years mortality – 8.3%
in the control group and 2.5% in the intervention group.

Perceptual and Physiological Responses to Training

Ben–Ari et al (14) examined at our laboratory the physiological
and perceptual (RPE) responses to very low and moderate intensity
training programs. Perceptual response was obtained using Borg's
scale (consisting of grades from 6 to 20, arranged as follows:
7 – very, very light; 9 – very light; 11 – 19 – very hard). Four
months of low intensity training showed significant ($p < 0.01$–0.o8)
decrease in HR, SBP and RPE at similar workloads. Additional
four months of moderate intensity resulted in further decrease

TABLE 3

HEART RATE (HR), RATE OF PERCEIVED EXERTION (RPE) SYSTOLIC BLOOD PRESSURE (SBP(AND SBP X HR PRODUCT BEFORE (T1), AFTER LOW INTENSITY (R2) AND MODERATE TRAINING (T3) IN CARDIAC PATIENTS WITH AND WITHOUT ANGINA PECTORIS

Work Loads–Watts		H.R/min			RPE			SBP mmHg			SBP x HR/100		
		T1	T2	T3	T1	T2	T3	T1	T2	T3	T1	T2	T3
1. The Group with Angina													
50W	Mean	102	97	100	10.5	10.3(b)	9.7	148	150(a)	131	149	145	130
	S.D.	16.5	17.	15.	1.2	1.1	2	12	5	11	19	54	27
			T1–T3(b)			T1–T3(b)			T1–T3(b)			T1–T3(b)	
75W	Mean	130(a)	117	112	14.3(a)	13	12.5	175	165	160	227(a)	183	184
	S.D.	17	22	24	1.1	2	3.5	15	15	19	40	61	42
			T1–T3(b)						T1–T3(b)			T1–T3(b)	
100W	Mean	137(b)	130	125	14(b)	13.5(a)	12	190	180	170	260(a)	232(a)	212
	S.D.	16.5	10	18	1.4	.3	1.4	9	0	13	23	11	51
			T1–T3(a)			T1–T3(a)			T1–T3(a)			T1–T3(a)	
2. Without Angina													
50W	Mean	110	106	105	10.4	10.4(b)	9.2	161	157	154	176	167	165
	S.D.	11	7.6	5.8	1.1	.78	2	17	12	13	44	14	35
75W	Mean	137	137	132	14(b)	13	13.5	190(b)	170	170	258(a)	232	230
	S.D.	8.3	12	14	1.4	.5	2	14	17	12	44	43	47
						T1–T3(a)			T1–T3(a)			T1–T3(b)	
100W	Mean	157	157	145	14.2	14	14	218	185	180	340	280	260
	S.D.	19	4.4	15	2.1	2.2		13	24	10	29	26	43
			T1–T3(b)						T1–T3(b)			T1–T3(a)	

3.Control Group

50W	Mean	103	102	103	12.2	12.1	12.5	150	155	160	152	153	160
	S.D.	8.0	11.3	13.	1.9	1.6	1.6	11	16	18	19	20	32
75W	Mean	127	127	128	13.5	14	14	160	170	150	205	210(a)	185
	S.D.	5	7	75	1.2	1.8	1.5	17	9	8	25	33	40
									T1–T3(b)				
100W	Mean	137	133	132	15	15	15.5	180	170	182	236	228	241
	S.D.	13.	11	11	1.6	1.6	1.5	19	20	19	32	13	30

Significance between tests is assigned as follows: a = $p > 0.01$, b = $p > 0.05$ between columns indicate differences between T1–T2 or T2–T3. Differences between T1–T3 is marked in rows.

in HR and RPE. Thus, in a well balanced, controlled program,
psychological factors play a major role, rather than physiological
changes, in the first part of cardiac rehabilitation involving
mostly low intensity programs. (see table 3).

DISCUSSION

    Physical training on selected patients with angina pectoris
can be accepted as a modality of therapy with the aim to improve
the physical capabilities of the patient. It has been demonstrated
repeatedly that physical training not only improves exercise
performance, but some data is available that myocardial oxygen
delivery may be improved. (15) The effect of training in these
patients depends on the reduction of MVO_2 at a given work
intensity suggested by the decrease of heart rate and systolic
blood pressure in well trained patients. Moreover we found that
in approximately 20.25% a higher angina pectoris threshold heart
rate and double product has been achieved after training. The
mechanism of these improvements are not quite clear.

    The following possibilities should be mentioned:

    (a) An increased maximal VO_2.

    (b) Enhanced oxygen supply.

    (c) Increased oxygen extraction.

    (d) Acceleration of collateral vessels.

    (e) A change in proximal steal.

    Not enough scientific evidence can be presented for most
of the aforementioned interpretations, nor is there any sufficient
evidence that other determinants of MVO_2 such as left ventricular
end-diastolic volume, myocardial contractility and left wall
thickness are affected directly by physical training. It is
however not impossible that there is an improved contractility
in response to physical training. Finally we should like to
point out another factor which in our opinion must be taken into
consideration. There is no doubt about the very beneficial
psychological effect of physical training in coronary patients.
As found in our laboratory there are significant changes in
perceptual responses after training, therefore it may be
possible that the subjective feeling of pain is decreased and
even ignored as a consequence of the reduced sensitivity to pain
in some patients and improved physical performance may be found.

    On the basis of our knowledge today the implementation of

carefully prepared and controlled physical training programs in well selected patients with angina pectoris can be considered as good medical practice.

References

1. J. J. Kellermann and I. Kariv, "Rehabilitation of coronary patients." Monography, Segal Press, 102 p., (1970).
2. J. J. Kellermann, B. Modan, S. Feldmann, I. Kariv. Return to work after myocardial infarction. Geriatrics, 23:151-156 (1968).
3. J. J. Kellermann. Rehabilitation of patients with coronary heart disease. Progress in Cardiovascular Diseases, 17: 303-328 (1975).
4. S. Holmberg, W. Serzysko, E. Varnauskas. Coronary circulation during heavy exercise in control subjects and patients with coronary heart disease. Acta Med. Scand. 190:465-480 (1971).
5. J. P. Clausen. Circulatory adjustments to dynamic exercise and effect of physical training in normal subject and in patients with coronary artery disease. Progress in Cardio-vascular Diseases. 18:459-495 (1976).
6. J. P. Clausen, O. A. Larsen, J. Trape-Jensen. Physical training in the management of coronary artery disease. Circulation, 40:143-154 (1969).
7. J.J.Kellermann. Exercise as preventive measure: A controversion in Kellermann J. J. and Denolin H. (eds.) Critical Evaluation of Cardiac Rehabilitation. Biblthca Cardiol. 36:30-36 Karger Basel (1977).
8. J. J. Kellermann. "Rehabilitation and secondary prevention in the context of comprehensive cardiovascular control programme at community level." Report of a W.H.O. meeting on comprehensive cardiovascular community control programmes. Edmonton, Alberta, Canada, November (1978).
9. J. J. Kellermann, E. Ben-Ari, M. Hayet, Ch. Lapidot, Y. Drory, and E. Fisman. Cardiocirculatory response to different types of training in patients with angina pectoris. Cardiology, 62:218-231 (1977).
10. E. Ben-Ari, J. J. Kellermann. The effect of prolonged intensive training on cardiorespiratory response in patients with angina pectoris. British Heart Journal. 40:1143-1148 (1978).
11. J. M. R. Detry. In: "Exercise Testing and Training in Coronary Heart Disease." H. E. Stenfert and B. V. Kroese ed., Leiden (1973).
12. P. O. Astrand, K. Rodahl. Textbook of Work Physiology, pp.373-430, McGraw-Hill, New York (1970).
13. M. Hayet, J. J. Kellermann. "Angina Pectoris Threshold Heart Rate as a prognostic sign." in Proc. of Int. Sym. on Exercise Testing and Training in Coronary Patients, E. Hirshhaut, ed., Caracas, (1979) (to be published).

14. E. Ben-Ari, J. J. Kellermann. "Perceptual and physiological response to training." (to be published).
15. D. R. Redwood, D. R. Rosing, S. E. Epstein. Circulatory and symptomatic effects of physical training in patients with coronary artery disease and angina pectoris. New England Journal of Medicine, 286:959-965 (1972).

PSYCHOLOGICAL ASPECTS OF CARDIAC REHABILITATION

Elizabeth L. Cay

Astley Ainslie Hospital
Edinburgh
Scotland, U.K.

HISTORICAL BACKGROUND

Psychological interest in ischaemic heart disease was initially almost entirely limited to the role of psychological factors in aetiology. By 1943 Dunbar had outlined a specific personality type that was said to be prone to develop the disease. Friedman and Rosenman developed this further with their definitions of personality type A, characterised by drive, ambition and impatience, which they reported was associated with an excess risk of coronary heart disease before the age of 60. Other workers have failed to confirm this and current opinion is that, as yet, there is no definitive evidence of the existence of "the coronary personality".

Much work has also been done on the role of antecedent stress as a risk factor since Selye published his early work in 1953. Levi and his co-workers in Stockholm have outlined the psychological pathways by which "stress" can influence blood clotting time, cardiac output, pulse rate, blood pressure and serum catecholamine levels and Rahe has examined the influence of emotionally charged life events immediately preceding the onset of acute myocardial infarction. More recently Theorell has published a series of studies on the influence of various aspects of the work environment (changes, conflicts and lack of appreciation by superiors) on healthy males and on the survivors of an infarction. But these workers are the first to admit that the pathway from psychosocial stresses to disease manifestation is complicated with whole areas still uncharted.

Towards the end of the nineteen fifties psychological interest became less preoccupied with problems of aetiology; papers began

to appear with the then revolutionary suggestion that psychological
factors were important in success or failure of treatment. This
was the consequence of the changing pattern in incidence and in
treatment of acute myocardial infarction. Not only was the incidence
of the disease increasing but the number of young people affected
grew rapidly. It was not enough that they survived the acute
infarct; they wanted life afterwards to be as near normal as
possible. The attitude of the medical profession was also changing.
The advantages of early mobilization were demonstrated by Levine
in 1952 and over the next few years studies in experimental animals
and in man showed that it was possible to improve physical
performance after myocardial infarction by exercise training. By
the end of the nineteen fifties exercise programmes for highly
selected patients were introduced. The need to evaluate this new
method of treating coronary patients prompted physicians and
cardiologists to examine their results. They demonstrated
improvement in physiological functioning, in working capacity, in
the proportion who returned to work and at the same time examined
critically those who failed to reach their estimated rehabilitation
potential. Causes for failure were not purely physical; a variety
of personal factors, socioeconomic problems and family and cultural
influences emerged. Precise identifications of psychosocial factors
was frequently not attempted and they were added together as
"adverse psychological influences".

     Psychologists and psychologically-orientated research workers
began to observe these aspects in more detail. Many of these
studies can be criticised on methodology. They were anecdotal with
little of no objective measurement, the group of patients selected
for study was illdefined or unrepresentative and many seemed to
ignore completely physical aspects such as severity, length of
time after the acute illness and whether or not there had been
a previous infarction. Methods of investigation which were suitable
for psychiatric illness were assumed to be equally relevant for
patients after myocardial infarction. Return to work was
assumed to be the goal of successful rehabilitation. Gradually,
however, it became apparent that there was growing agreement on
the psychological factors that were important in outcome.

a)   Emotional reaction to the illness. Anxiety and fear were
common and Wynn described considerable unwarranted emotional
distress in patients after a heart attack. Anxiety if severe
might well be the main reason for failure to return to work.
Unrelieved depression with resulting loss of confidence and
sense of insecurity was also a reason for failure.

b)   Personality traits were important rather than a specific
personality type. The inadequate, overdependent individual was
likely to be satisfied with the "sick" role. The methods of
coping with stress which the individual had developed over the

years determined how he coped with ischaemic heart disease.

These personal attitudes were influenced by a number of
environmental factors; attitudes to heart disease prevalent in his
culture; the attitudes of his family, his age, social class
which determined his type of employment, the reactions of fellow
workers and employers to the individual who has had a myocardial
infarction and the socioeconomic conditions in his country at the
time of his illness.

Comprehensive Rehabilitation

Within the last decade there has been a significant change
in the concept of cardiac rehabilitation. Communication has been
increasing between physically orientated medical practitioners and
their psychologically trained colleagues. The idea of comprehensive
rehabilitation with its goal the development of a programme to
improve the patient's capacity for physical work and his emotional
wellbeing has gained general acceptance. Cardiac centres in various
countries have developed programmes where this team approach is
practised and their results are beginning to suggest that considerable improvement in outcome is feasible. Rehabilitated patients
return to work earlier and function more efficiently than do non-
rehabilitated patients. Hospital based studies suggest that about
80% of survivors following an infarct eventually return to work
without special measures. The proportion returning by three
months is variable but often is in the order of 40-50%. This can
be contrasted with figures from rehabilitation orientated centres
where 80-90% are back by this time.

This change in treatment is reflected in research trends over
the past few years. There has been a distinct move towards
investigation by a research team so that physical, psychological
and social variables are examined in the same group of patients
enabling interactions between them to be studied. The emotional
reactions of the patient to his illness have received considerable
attention. There is evidence now concerning the "natural history"
of his reactions from the onset of pain, throughout hospitalization
and during gradually increasing physical activity until he can
return to work and resume former leisure activities. The influence
of family attitudes has been studied and the effect of a myocardial
infarction on individual roles within the family, on the family
structure, on sexual functioning and in social networks examined.
Much work has been concerned with the psychological impact on the patient of physical methods of treatment. New techniques to measure
psychological variables have been described and efforts are being made
to improve the identification of those patients who will find it difficult to return to an active life. The advantages and disadvantages of
various psychological methods of treatment are currently being critically assessed.

NATURAL HISTORY

Naughton's view that rehabilitation begins from the onset of
the acute illness is widely accepted today, although it caused
controversy when it was expressed in 1967. It can be divided into
three stages depending on the physical state of the patient;
Stage I (Acute Phase), Stage II (Convalescent Phase) and Stage III
(Post-convalescent or Maintenance Phase). Psychological reactions
to the illness and their appropriate care will be different at each
stage and parallel the change in physical state.

Psychological reactions during the acute phase

Fear and anxiety occur most commonly. This may be fear of
death, of reinfarction or loss of the established pattern of
living. Continuing symptoms, breathlessness and chest pain, may
also increase anxiety. Hackett has shown that a less obvious
symptom which may provoke anxiety is weakness, particularly in young
previously healthy men. Patients often regard weakness as proving
that the illness is irreversible or that heart damage is permanent.
Methods of treatment may provoke anxiety; the dash to hospital,
admission to a coronary care unit, immobilization in bed and dependency on others. The attitude of the physician is all important;
Hellerstein has shown that anxious doctors have anxious patients.

Not all patients present a manifest anxiety picture. They
may appear overdependent, demanding immediate attention and care.
Hostility may occur when various external sources including the
physician may be blamed for the illness, hypochondriasis with
overconcern with bodily functions or denial of the illness with
disregard of sensible medical advice. Some patients may use their
illness as a solution for premorbid neurotic problems. If anxiety
is unrelieved depression may be obvious, particularly after a
second infarction. Hackett has reported that this is reactive in
nature and rarely assumes psychotic proportions. In his experience
anxiety occurs early, usually on the first or second day, while
depression has its highest incidence on the third day after onset
of physical symptoms. The depressed patient appears sad. dis-
interested and listless, is slow of speech and despondent about the
future; he foresees reinfaction, reduced earning power, sexual
incompetence, invalidism and premature old age. Various studies
have examined the frequency of such emotional reactions during the
acute phase.

Their results are not strictly comparable in that the groups
under scrutiny differ diagnostically, in the method used to estimate
disturbance (clinical interview and/or questionnaire) and in the
length of time after onset when the measurements were made. But
they agree that between half and threequarters of patients
immediately after an infarction are anxious and depressed.

	Number of Patients	Emotional Disturbance		Time of Assessment (Days)
HACKETT (1974) ET AL	36	Anxiety 30% Mild 40% Moderate 6% Severe	Depression 35% Mild 36% Moderate 6% Severe	1-3
CAY ET AL (1972)	131	Emotional Upset 61%	Significant Upset - 1st MI 30% " " subseq MI 42%	8-10
CAY ET AL (1976)	197	29% Significant Anxiety	20% Significant Depression	5-8
STERN ET AL (1977)	63	42% Anxious 19% Moderate/Severe	29% Depressed 18% Moderate/Severe	6

Fig.1. Emotional reaction to myocardial infarction - acute phase.

These reactions are independent of the physical severity of the illness, but are influenced by the patient's premorbid personality, the methods of coping with stress which he has developed over the years, by his previous experience, by attitudes to heart disease in his culture and by existing environmental problems, especially those connected with work. Emotional reactions to a heart attack are not static but involve a continuous process of readjustment by the patient.

	1st MI	Subsequent MI	Ischaemia (No previous MI)	Ischaemia (Previous MI)
Number of Patients	99	30	47	27
Physical Severity				
Peel Index	12.9	21.2	7.1	13.6
Norris Index	5.7	6.7	2.8	3.9
Anxiety (Cattell 8 - Parallel Form)				
Mean Anxiety Score	5.8	4.9	5.9	5.4

Anxiety and Peel Index r = -0.03   Anxiety and Norris Index r = -0.06

Fig.2. Initial reaction to a heart attack in relation to physical severity.

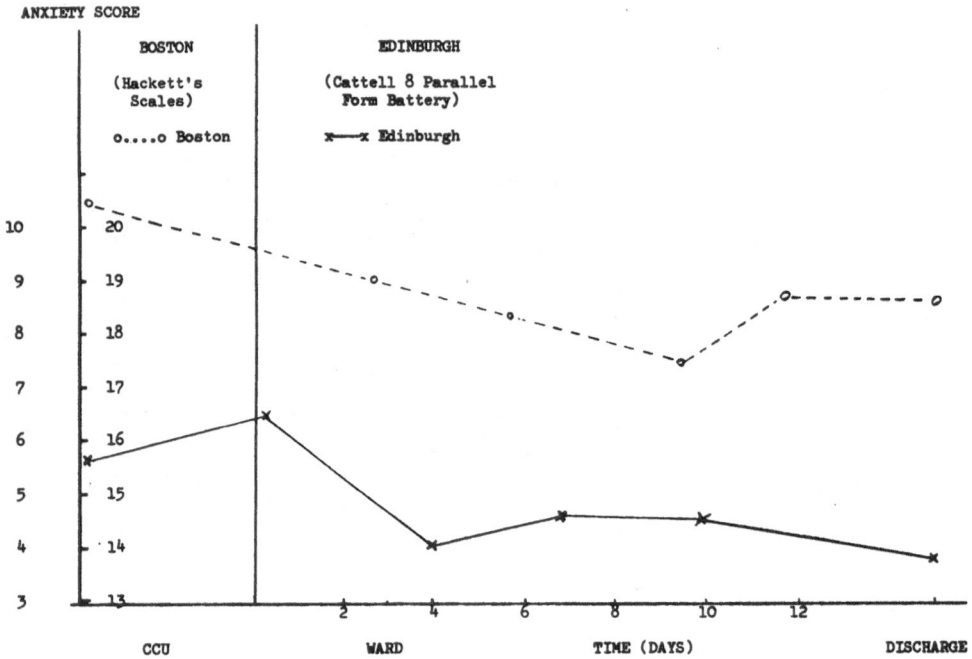

Figure 3.   Anxiety after a heart attack

      The Boston patients who were initially very anxious became
progressively less so until discharge from hospital became imminent.
On the other hand, the Edinburgh patients were more anxious
immediately after transfer from the Coronary Care Unit to the
medical ward and showed very little anxiety in the 24 hours before
discharge suggesting that the excitement of going home temporarily
dispelled their worries and fears. However, the findings from
Boston and Edinburgh concur in demonstrating relatively
unchanging levels of anxiety in the middle portion of time spent in
hospital.

      The effect of family attitudes is extremely important. During
the acute illness the wife's anxiety may be greater than that of
her husband.

Psychological reactions during convalescence

      During this phase there is steadily increasing physical
activity designed to provide the patient with tangible evidence of
return to normal health. There are considerable psychological

hazards for the patient in his efforts to return to normal daily
life and he seldom foresees them. With greater activity there may
be increased appreciation of physical limitations and common
complaints at this stage are weakness and tiredness. There is a
tendency to interpret such symptoms as evidence of deterioration
in cardiac function and as a result depression and anxiety may
persist or appear in the first month of convalenscence. The lack
of structure in the lives of those accustomed to a busy existence
results in boredom, frustration and loss of confidence. Insomnia
is common and as a result he may be irritable and quick to take
offence and may seek to prolong his invalid role and impose
excessive demands on his family. Such reactions are common and
persistent. Cay et al found that 51% of their patients were
anxious or depressed four months after their infarct and 56%
at one year. Stern et al found 73% of those depressed immediately
after infarction remained so throughout follow up and Singh et al
found 34% of patients were depressed or anxious in the two years
following an infarct.

Outcome in these disturbed patients was poor.

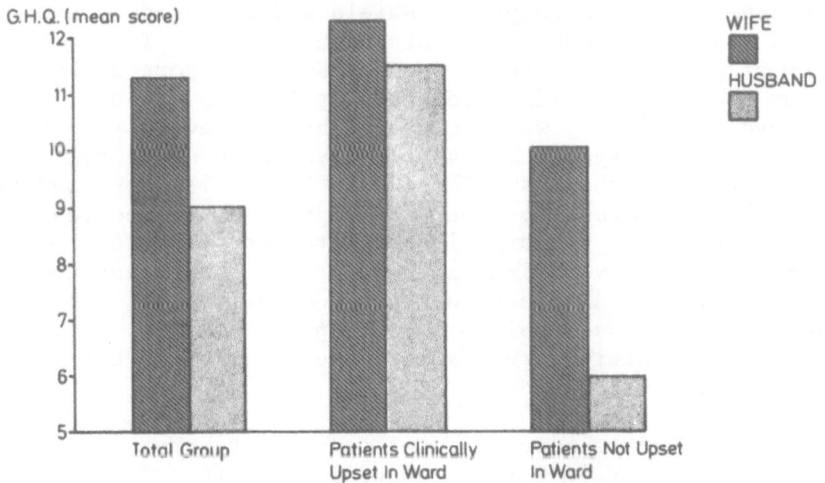

Fig. 4. Wives' anxiety while husband in hospital with a first
Myocardial Infarction. (General questionnaire)

EMOTIONAL UPSET 5-8 days after MI	RETURN TO FULL ACTIVITY BY 4/12	RETURN TO FULL ACTIVITY WITHIN 1 yr
Absent	52%	88%
Present	36%	31%

Fig.5. Return to work related to initial reaction to MI.

Fewer returned to work and of those who did return few
regained their previous level of activity even after prolonged
convalescence. Return to work does not always depend on physical
severity of the infarction; in Goble's series, in 40% reasons
for failure to return to work were psychological without any
somatic justification and Nagle reported that non-cardiac causes
of invalidism were just as important as cardiac causes in failure
to earn a living.

As a result of the patient's uncertainties, problems
connected with work and possible financial stringencies, his wife
may be uncertain how to cope with the situation and be anxious
whether her attitude is promoting or retarding rehabilitation. If
her anxiety is exaggerated and disproportionate to the patient's
current disability her attempts to shield and overprotect him will
be resented and may provoke outbursts of hostility. In a comparative study of patients and their spouses Ruskin reported that
neuroticism scores were higher for patient than for spouse, but
that her level of anxiety was influenced by the severity of her
husband's illness. Mayou found 42% of wives were depressed two
months after their husband's infarct with 30% still depressed at a
year. Predictive factors for the wife's progress at one year were
her mental state, work satisfaction, marital satisfaction and a
previous history of psychiatric illness. It is important that
the whole family should adjust to the new situation; if the family
is experiencing serious problems in interpersonal life, social
and economic difficulties, the patient's chances of successful
rehabilitation are decreased.

Anxiety related to resumption of sexual intercourse may
cause considerable strain between husband and wife. Tuttle found
that two thirds of his patients after an infarct reported a marked
and lasting reduction in the frequency of intercourse as a result

of lack of information and fear. Several studies have examined the physicological effect of sexual activity on the cardiovascular system in young healthy adults but Hellerstein and Friedman measured this for the first time in middle-aged males after an infarct, and demonstrated that the mean maxium heart rate during intercourse with their wives was less than during daily work activity. The frequency of death during intercourse, a repeated source of anxiety, was investigated by Ueno. He found that death in 34 out of 5,559 cases of sudden death was precipitated by sexual activity but in the great majority of cases death occurred during intercourse with other than an "established" marital or sexual partner in a secretive encounter in a hotel rather than in the privacy of one's home.

During convalescence other external factors influence the individual's emotional reactions. Problems connected with return to work are paramount. The attitudes of his workmates may increase his fear that physically he may not be able to cope especially if he has residual angina or breathlessness. The family's economic circumstances will have significant bearing on an early return to work particularly if he is self-employed while continuation of salary during illness and social security benefits will have the reverse effect. Serious problems may arise when the patient wants to return to work but cannot for legal or other reasons. Success in changing a job depends on many things such as employers' prejudice, the patient's educational and vocational skills and the socio-economic situation. It has been shown that an individual's work record after an infarct compares favourably with that of his fellow-employees. As might be expected, professional and managerial workers find it easier to earn their living after a heart attach than do those with semi-skilled or unskilled jobs.

Psychological reactions during maintenance phase

By the beginning of this stage most individuals should be at a high level of physical and psychological recovery. Return to work is a significant event for the patient and his family who may view it with apprehension. The doctor should re-emphasise that return to work is not dangerous and that a feeling of weakness and tiredness during the introductory period is common and a passing phenomenon. Rehabilitation after myocardial infarction involves considerable re-education as regards the continuing value of physical fitness, the avoidance of risk factors and the cultivation of hobbies and interests. Advantages gained during the acute and convalescent phases will be lost if the individual later slips back into previous bad habits. The detrimental effect of restrictive and over-protective attitudes is at least as great from now on as it was earlier.

Social Class	Working By 4 Months	Average Time To Return (Days)
I and II (professional, managerial)	95%	52
III (skilled)	64%	92
IV (semi-skilled)	60%	106
V (unskilled)	55%	95

Fig. 6. Social class of patient in relation to return to work.

The post-arrest patient

        Some years ago the first reports were published describing
the quality of life after surviving cardiac arrest. They made
depressing reading. The incidence of depression, nightmares and
chronic anxiety was high. The survivors complained of "being
different from other people". These observations have not been a
feature of later studies and there now seems to be little or no
psychological sequelae of cardiac arrest. The reasons for this
may lie in the way in which the patient learns that he has arrested.
In the beginning there was no uniform policy and often the wife
or a relative informed the patient, usually in highly dramatic
terms. Doctors, probably unsure themselves, usually remained
silent. Since the experience was unique to doctor and patient
alike, distortion, exaggeration and misinformation accrued. Dobson
et al followed a series who survived cardiac arrest for some years.
They commented on the absence of emotional upset and showed that
ventricular fibrillation, by itself, did not adversely affect the
patient's prognosis. They advised that the patient should be told
of his arrest by the doctor within twenty four hours of the
event, that its routine nature be emphasised and that the patient
and his family should be informed that the future was not more
gloomy because of it. Nine out of ten patients do not remember
much of the arrest though the patient who has had more than one is
likely to be aware of it. A few patients do,however, remain alert

and conscious throughout. They may complain about the pain they
suffered but they do not appear to be more anxious than the majority
who remember little or nothing.

Psychological aspects of coronary bypass surgery

The advent of coronary bypass surgery was a spectacular step
in the treatment of ischaemic heart disease and the number of
patients being operated on has increased rapidly over the past few
years. Improvement in angina pectoris following operation occurs
in about 90%, with complete relief of symptoms in about two thirds
of the patients. Symptomatic improvement is thus often sufficient
to allow patients to return to work. However, a combination of
social, economic and psychological factors may prevent successfull
rehabilitation. The longer the period of inactivity before surgery
the less likely is a return to work.

Very little is as yet known about the incidence of
psychological problems and their effects on the patient after
coronary bypass surgery. In one of the very few studies to discuss
psychological problems Rabiner and Willner examined 51 patients
during the immediate post operative period in hospital and at
follow up about eighteen months later, and compared their progress
with 46 patients undergoing cardiac valvular surgery. The incidence
of post-operative psychiatric symptoms was 16% in the bypass group
and 41% in the valvular surgical patients. At follow-up there was
no significant difference between the two groups, 15% of the bypass
patients having symptoms and 31% of the others. Of those with
psychiatric symptoms in the bypass group, 3 were depressed, 2
were depressed with evidence of organic brain damage and 2 had
evidence of organic brain damage alone. There was no indication
that patients who developed psychiatric symptoms in hospital were
likely to have symptoms at follow up,suggesting that the delirious
patients tend to recover spontaneously. Pre-operative psychological
morbidity was significantly related to symptoms at follow up; it
should be possible, therefore, to identify the "psychological bad
risks" before operation. Obviously more work on these aspects must
be done before this can be said with any certainty.

ASSESSMENT OF THE PATIENT

It is important to stress that psychological assessment is
part of total patient care and must be closely allied to an
accurate assessment of physical state. The methods of examining
the patient which can be carried out at an early stage will depend
on severity of the infarction, the degree of recovery, presence
of complications and other medical illnesses. Later on, the
interplay of residual disability (angina or breathlessness),
physical working capacity, psychological morbidity and various
social factors will influence the patient's rehabilitation potential.

At each stage of illness the psychological assessment must include
(1) an assessment of those factors within the patient which promote
or hinder rehabilitation and (2) an assessment of factors in the
patient's environment at home, at work, or in the pursuit of his
leisure activities which will influence rehabilitation.

Aims of Assessment

The physician has two aims in his assessment of his patient:
diagnosis and prediction. Diagnosis of the individual's
psychological reactions to the acute stress situation and the
methods of defence which he mobilises to help him to cope with
it allows the physician to predict how successful his patient will
be in returning to an active productive life. Using this information
he can then treat his patient rationally.

It is important to see the spouse separately; the patient may
not be telling the truth and the wife herself may need guidance
and treatment.

Guide lines for assessment

Awareness by the physician that his patient after a heart attack
is likely to be anxious or depressed and that he may have social
problems is the first step in positive identification of these
aspects of patient care. It would seem that the physician's attitude
and the image he conveys is one of the most potent factors in
combatting anxiety and preventing iatrogenic disease. Authors have
stressed the importance of the optimistic approach though Mendel
feels that this is too simple; he maintains that the physician must
strike the balance between the powerful protecting figure and one
who appreciates the situation realistically. This is particularly
important in patients who have shown evidence before the infarction
of inability to cope with other stresses of adult like. Indicators
of this are poor work records, previous psychiatric history,
excessive invalidism after other illnesses, a poor martial relationship and pre-existing financial problems. The reasons why the
patient is reacting badly are as important as diagnosis of
disturbance. They determine the method of treatment which may be
relatively simple involving only minor adjustments at work, or
prolonged and difficult if emotional disturbance is arising on
the basis of premorbid personality traits which may cause the
individual to seek to prolong the invalid role.

Hackett has pointed out that anxiety may be difficult to
identify because patients consciously or unconsciously deny it.
There has been considerable controversy on the role of denial in
cardiac rehabilitation. Some authors feel that denial hinders
adjustment because it prevents the patient's objective
assessment of the situation. This was supported by Ruskin's finding

that the aware and cautious patient improves most on follow up,
co-operates best with his medical advisors and returns to work
readily. Other workers have shown that denial, as a belief in the
"self" without disease, promotes rehabilitation. This is supported
by recent work by the Boston group. They found that moderate denial
may be associated with decreased morbidity and mortality after
infarction and that it is the small proportion of minimal deniers
who are likely to remain maladjusted.

Methods of assessment

Many methods have been used in research to estimate level of
anxiety, depression, denial, personality traits and motivation.
Psychologists have used a combination of interview, projective tests
and questionnaires. In an international survey in 1970,
Fisher found that the most commonly used method of assessment was
the interview followed by a variety of projective tests.
Questionnaires were less popular and tended to be confined to the
two personality inventories most in vogue at that time, the MMPI and
the 16PF. They were unsuitable for the non-psychologically trained
physician to administer and interpret, while others, originally
developed for neurotic patients, were not very relevant to patients
after a myocardial infarction. They reflected the need at that
time for maximum information, were very long and thus quite unsuited
to routine clinical practice. Recently research workers have
tended to use questionnaires rather than projective tests in the
quest for objective hard data. These tests have been much shorter
and a number have come into use which were originally developed
to estimate disturbance in a "normal" population. Other workers
have concentrated on developing specific scales to estimate upset
in the cardiac patient.

The importance of predicting on psychosocial grounds success
or failure in rehabilitation has led to considerable efforts to
find measures to estimate this. Rumbaugh in the mid sixties
developed a questionnaire of 160 items for predicting the adjustment
of the cardiac patient to his illness and his subsequent return to
work. Later, Josten produced his "subjective load" questionnaire,
measuring the degree to which the patient is occupied with his
illness and the problems created by it. Scores correlated well with
physical complaints and with psychiatric ratings of emotional
problems and differentiated between those who achieved various
levels of subsequent activity at work. Other measurements have
been shown to predict outcome; patient performance in a sheltered
workshop, breath holding time and preception of instructions by
the medical staff. At present several workers are concentrating
on the important task of producing a simple, screening method for
routine clinical use to predict those likely to have problems in
rehabilitation. Promising scales in this area are those of
Schiller and Hoffman though both have their shortcomings.

```
            8-PARALLEL FORM ANXIETY BATTERY    -    CATTELL

                    (1960)    -    ANXIETY


            NEUROTICISM SCORE QUESTIONNAIRE    -    CATTELL

                    (1965)    -    EMOTIONAL UPSET


            GENERAL HEALTH QUESTIONNAIRE    -    GOLDBERG

                    (1970)    -    EMOTIONAL UPSET


            STAI - SPIELBERGER (1970)    -    ANXIETY

                          ―――――


            HACKETT'S SCALES    -    ANXIETY

                                    DEPRESSION

                                    DENIAL
```

Fig. 7.   Questionnaires to estimate emotional disturbance.


```
    PHYSICAL SEVERITY - PEEL INDEX          ⎤
                                            ⎥  PHYSICIAN
    AGE                                     ⎦


    ANXIETY ON TRANSFER FROM CCU            ⎤

    ANXIETY IN WARD                         ⎥

    SYMPTOM SIGN INVENTORY (EMOTIONAL UPSET) ⎥  QUESTIONNAIRE

    EXTRA PUNITIVENESS                      ⎥

    INTRA PUNITIVENESS                      ⎦


    PSYCHOLOGICAL REACTION (ANXIETY,        ⎤
                        DEPRESSION)         ⎥  PSYCHIATRIST
    PERSONALITY RESOURCES (COPING)          ⎦
```

Fig. 8.   Assessment of patient immediately after a myocardial
          infarction.

To date the criterion of successful rehabilitation has usually been return to work. Recent thinking is that this is much too narrow and that an estimate of the individual's quality of life must be included. Andrews and Withey have developed a questionnaire to assess quality of life in an American population and this has been used to gather normative data on a British population. There is need now to assess this in various clinical groups but the importance of this recent work is to indicate that "quality of life" can be measured.

The whole area of predicting outcome after a myocardial infarction is fraught with difficulty. Recently a group in Edinburgh have examined the usefulness of various methods of assessing the patient during his stay in hospital in predicting outcome one year later.

The physician's assessment of physical severity of the attack and readily available data such as age; questionnaire scores on aspects of personality and emotional reactions in hospital; and clinical assessments requiring an interview by a trained psychiatrist were considered.

The outcome measures included survival or not, the physician's estimate of residual disability, the psychiatrist's examination of psychological morbidity, social outcome and the patient's own reported problems in various areas.

Physical outcome and indeed the patient's survival for a year were not predictable from the available information. Prospects of working as well as before his infarct and psychiatric morbidity could be foreseen, as were those who considered that they were physically disabled with difficulty in earning their living and coping with their jobs and finances. Using regression analysis it was possible to estimate the contribution which each of the measurements in the ward made to those aspects of outcome which were predictable.

As might be expected, the severity of the heart attack was important in returning to work. The patient's own estimate of disability one year later depended on the severity of infarct but equally important was his personality resources (how he had learned to cope with problems). Those who had reacted badly in the beginning tended to consider themselves disabled. Problems in working again depended on severity personality and inversely with age; the younger patients having more problems than the older ones. Those who reacted badly in the beginning were still those anxious and depressed one year later.

But in general the prediction is not particularly good when the overall contribution that these initial estimates make is considered. It may be that one year is too long. Perhaps now

```
ALIVE/DEAD

PHYSICIAN            ANGINA, BREATHLESS, CCF, ISCHAEMIC ATTACKS

PSYCHIATRIST         PSYCHOLOGICAL SYMPTOMS, CHANGE IN SYMPTOMS

SOCIAL OUTCOME       JOB CHANGE, SOCIAL STATE, SMOKING

PATIENT  -  REPORTED DIFFICULTIES;  PHYSICAL
                                    WORK
                                    FINANCIAL
                                    MARITAL/FAMILY
```

Fig. 9. Outcome one year after a myocardial infarction.

	R	R^2	F RATIO	P LEVEL
ALIVE/DEAD	.36	.13	1.60	NS
ANGINA	.37	.13	1.05	NS
BREATHLESSNESS	.34	.11	1.00	NS
CCF	.34	.11	0.88	NS
ISCHAEMIC ATTACKS	.36	.13	1.01	NS
JOB CHANGE	.51	.26	2.51	.025*
SOCIAL STATE	.63	.18	1.51	NS
SMOKING	.39	.15	1.44	NS
PHYSICAL DIFFICULTIES	.50	.25	2.28	.05*
WORK "	.63	.40	3.52	.01*
FINANCIAL "	.52	.27	2.59	.025*
HOME "	.25	.06	0.68	NS
PSYCHOLOGICAL SYMPTOMS	.51	.26	2.36	.025*
CHANGE IN SYMPTOMS	.68	.47	6.02	.001*

Fig. 10. Prediction of outcome 1 year after myocardial infarction from information in ward.

OUTCOME	CONTRIBUTING VARIABLE	PORTION ADDED TO CORRELATION (%)	F RATIO	P LEVEL
JOB CHANGE	PEEL INDEX	12	10.84	.01
	SSI	4	3.83	NS
	WARD ANXIETY	3	3.16	NS
PHYSICAL DIFFICULTIES	PEEL INDEX	5	4.20	.05
	TRANSFER ANXIETY	6	4.99	.05
	PERSONALITY RESOURCES	9	7.86	.01
WORK DIFFICULTIES	PEEL	10	8.23	.01
	−AGE	5	4.21	.05
	EXTRA P	7	5.94	.025
	PERSONALITY RESOURCES	12	10.1	.01
FINANCIAL DIFFICULTIES	−AGE	4	3.63	NS
	PERSONALITY RESOURCES	8	7.02	.025
PSYCHOLOGICAL SYMPTOMS	TRANSFER ANXIETY	10	8.74	.01
	EXTRA P	2	2.09	NS
	PERSONALITY RESOURCES	7	5.69	.025
CHANGE IN PSYCHOLOGICAL SYMPTOMS	WARD ANXIETY	3	3.23	NS
	INTRA P	2	2.62	NS
	SYMPTOMS IN WARD	28	32.77	.001
	PERSONALITY RESOURCES	5	5.58	.025

Fig. 11. Variables assessed in ward making significant prediction of outcome one year after a myocardial infarction.

attention should be focussed on the importance of initial estimates in predicting outcome in the short term i.e. in identifying those who require special measures to achieve successful rehabilitation.

For the physician, faced with the task of assessing his patient, there is at present no one simple screening test. He knows that several psychosocial factors are important in predicting which of his patients will do well and which will do badly. The clinical interview is the most reliable method at the moment to obtain the information he needs. At a meeting in 1976 of the Council on Rehabilitation, International Society of Cardiology a working group outlined the format of a semi-structured interview designed to help the physician in his assessment. Psychosocial factors included in the interview were anxiety, depression, denial, work problems, family problems including sexual activity, problems involving leisure activities and problems in complying with medical advice. Its purpose was screening for the presence of psychosocial problems, assessing their severity and judging whether or not specialist advice should be sought.

Treatment

    Rehabilitation should not be considered an isolated therapeutic
acitivity but rather as one of the facets of care of the whole
patient. It can be stressed that the great majority of patients
with psychosocial problems can be treated by the physician involved
in their physical care. Only a minority with severe disturbance
or grave social problems will require specialist treatment,
possibly about 20% of patients.

Treatment during the acute phase

    Psychologically, the patient's first point of contact with the
medical profession after onset of the acute symptoms is critical
because it is his introduction to the setting of care. It is usually
with his medical practitioner or hospital casualty doctor. Prompt
attendance with speedy relief of pain by sedatives and analgesics
accompanied by an attitude of positive encouragement will go far to
dispel initial anxiety. Patients appreciate being told the truth
directly and matter-of-factly and mention of discharge within a few
weeks even at this stage often serves as a reassuring yardstick for
the patient in a new frightening world full of uncertainties. It is
important to see the relatives as soon as possible to explain the
nature of the illness and to outline the treatment in hospital.

    The modern approach is to admit to a Coronary Care Unit at the
earliest possible moment all patients with suspected myocardial
infarction to deal with serious complications, especially arrhythmias.
Such emergency admission may in itself present psychological problems
as the speed of events gives the patient little time to adjust and
emphasise to him and his family that he is seriously ill. The
Coronary Care Unit can, however, be a potent source of reassurance.

    Provided staff are aware that patients are likely to be anxious
or depressed and supportive measures given, such as explanation
of the monitoring equipment and tranquillizers to sedate the patient
and reduce anxiety, experience is now that patients are reassured
by their stay in these specialized units. Transfer from the unit
is not a psychological hazard provided that the patient knows from
the time of admission that his stay is only for a short time, until
his heart has stabilized and no longer requires monitoring.

    There is not an excess of anxiety in those who were sorry to
leave the CCU within 24 hours of their stay in the ward.

    Fear and anxiety may stem from the patient's inadequate
knowledge of the natural history of the disease and its treatment.

1   INITIAL PSYCHOLOGICAL REACTIONS

    (when clinical state of patient is stable in CCU)

    Anxiety, depression, denial

2   PSYCHOSOCIAL STATE IN HOSPITAL

    Anxiety, depression, denial

    Social items: occupation, educational level, problems in

    returning to work, family problems

Fig. 12(a).   Outline of psychosocial assessment of patient after
               myocardial infarction.

3   PSYCHOSOCIAL STATE AFTER DISCHARGE (approx 2 weeks)

    Anxiety, depression, denial

    Social items: attitudes of employer and family, work problems

    family problems, compliance with medical advice, attitude

    towards a rehabilitation programme.

4   EVALUATION OF OUTCOME (when the majority should have returned

    to work)

    Anxiety, depression, denial

    Work items: return to work, level of activity, reasons for

    failure to return, finances, attitudes about working.

    Social items: effect on family, leisure activities, compliance

    with medical advice.

Fig. 12(b).   Outline of psychosocial assessment of patient after
               myocardial infaction.

There is some debate whether single rooms are better than two
or four-bedded rooms in a CCU. Companionship is an argument in
favour of the latter while fear of witnessing a cariac arrest is
cited by those who favour single rooms. Studies have shown that
patients in a CCU rarely complain of being lonely; many like
privacy to adjust to having a heart attack.

Witnessing a cardiac arrest was found by Hackett to have
frightened only 20% of his patients, who seemed to be reassured
by the speed and efficiency of the medical and nursing staff.
Lack of identification with the victim particularly if he died was
the usual response and this was deliberately fostered by the staff
who explained that the deceased's heart was much worse than that of
the other patients in the unit. In spite of this, requests for
tranquillizers, sedatives and analgesics in the unit rise immediately
following an arrest and patients who had witnessed an arrest said
they would prefer a single room should they require readmission. It
appears that anxiety provoked by witnessing a cardiac arrest may be
greater than the patient admits.

Transition to the medical ward, provided that simple measures
to allay anxiety, such as explanation, reassurance and perhaps some
increase in sedation are taken, is viewed as a tangible sign of
progress. Early mobilization decreases anxiety and depression.
A calm competent staff who take emergencies in their stride and
explain to the patient what they are doing and what is the next
stage in treatment are the most potent weapon against this. They
should have rehabilitation in mind from the very beginning and the
fact that the great majority of patients do return to work and to
an active life should be stressed even in the CCU. Patients and
their relatives vary in educational level and anxiety decreases
understanding. It is important that explanations are given in
terms that they can understand and are repeated at frequent
intervals. Time to allow patients and relatives to ask questions
is not wasted.

Some centres start a programme of physical conditioning about the
third day of illness. Reports to date indicate that emotional
disturbance is much less when the patient is thus actively engaged.
He feels that he is taking part in his own recovery and gains in
confidence from the realization that physical activity under careful
supervision is not only possible but safe. Equally important, his
family have concrete evidence of his increasing physical abilities.

REACTION	FIRST M.I. %	SUBSEQUENT M.I. %	NO M.I., NO HISTORY M.I. %	NO M.I. PREVIOUS M.I. %	TOTAL %
Reassured)	90	80	81	67	83
Dependent)	3	10	4	7	5
Indifferent	5	3	13	11	7
Not reassured	2	7	2	15	5
	n = 99	n = 30	n = 47	n = 27	n = 203

Fig. 13. Reaction to the C.C.U.

Reaction on Discharge from C.C.U.	Mean Anxiety Score			
	First MI	Subsequent MI	No MI, no history MI	No MI, previous MI
Glad	6.0	5.0	5.8	5.5
Sorry	5.5	4.7	5.8	6.0
Indifferent	6.0	-	6.4	3.0

Fig. 14. Level of anxiety on day after transfer from the C.C.U. in relation to reaction on discharge.

REASON	NO. OF PATIENTS %
Staff efficiency	91
Continuous monitoring	84
Individual care	70
Privacy of single room	51
Frequent visiting by relatives	37

(* more than one reason given by many patients)

Fig. 15. Reasons given by patients for reassurance in the C.C.U.

With decrease in cardiac symptoms and improving physical well-being, the patient, in order to allay anxiety, wants to discuss the nature of his illness, the rational of treatment and the prognosis especially regarding his future capacity for work. From his assessment of the patient and his family and his knowledge of the severity of the attack the physician can judge how much to tell the patient. His aim is to minimize anxiety, to help the patient to set up some norms for the future and to reduce the ambiguity and uncertainty induced by the sudden onset of illness. Enlightened optimism is the keynote of the rehabilitation programme. An attitude of encouragement by the doctor is essential. He should try to explain the nature of the heart attack in terms which the patient can understand. If the individual asks about his chances of dying and recurrence the doctor can emphasize the hopeful and positive aspects of the illness without minimizing the risks. Ample time should be allowed for the patient to ask questions and to correct false impressions. It may be helpful to quote the later achievements of well-known people who have had heart attacks. At an early stage the doctor should encourage discussion about return to work. The family should be included in these discussions so that the adverse effects of the over-protection by his relatives can be avoided.

Though a programme of increasing activity and education of the patient is the best antidote for emotional disturbance, tranquillizers, especially the benzodiazepines which do not have

hypotensive side effects, have a definite place in the management
of anxiety. Tricyclic antidepressants have been reported as
causing cardiac arrhythmias and possible sudden death so their use
should be avoided if at all possible. The monoamine oxidase
inhibitors can cause fatal hypertensive crises if a tyramine-free
diet is not adhered to, so are seldom used in patients with
cardiovascular disease.

Patients who have been identified as having environmental
problems connected with work or within the family should receive
special attention. Physical state will determine how much can be
achieved at this relatively early stage but the aim should be
that the patient can leave hospital with the knowledge that help
to overcome such difficulties is already begun.

In recent years the period of hospitalization after an infarct
has been progressively shortened. In many countries the average
stay in hospital is now 10 to 14 days. While this has undoubted
psychological benefits it does require that preparation of patient
and family for return home becomes very important. In a proportion
of patients the impending loss of security implicit in discharge
can increase anxiety in the day or two before returning home. Overt
evidence that the patient is physically capable of, for example,
climbing the stairs to his flat and precise instructions about
gradually increasing his physical activity at home with advice about
avoidance of risk factors and drug regimes are necessary.
Recognizing that patients may be worried and anxious, some centres
have instituted regimes whereby an individual who has been involved
with the patient and his family from the beginning of his illness
remains in contact, if only by telephone, and available to deal with
problems as they arise.

The general principles of comprehensive rehabilitation are the
same irrespective of the actual way in which it is implemented.
The diverse nature of problems encountered has led in many hospitals
to the formation of a rehabilitation team, each member contributing
his own special skills depending on the individual's needs. The
doctor prescribes the physical programme which is carried out by the
physiotherapist. Nurses, psychologists, social workers and
occupational therapists have been variously used to permit free
discussion with the patient and his wife. Treatment can be on an
individual basis but groups are increasingly being formed in many
centres.

Treatment during the convalescent phase

Management of the patient is the same as for the acute phase.
Explanation to the patient and his family is essential to prepare
him to accept that feeling weak, fearful and uncertain is common
and almost a normal reaction during early convalescence. A wife

should be warned against totally supressing annoyance and impatience
towards her husband. The psychological advantages of exercise
testing followed by a definitive programme of physical rehabilitation
cannot be underestimated but if such programmes are not available
the patient and his wife should have a clear prescription from his
doctor of a gradual increase of physical activity. Vague advice
"to take things easily" must be avoided as it is open to wide
variations in individual interpretation. Strained marital
relationships may arise from uncertainties about the advisability
of resuming sexual intercourse and husband and wife should be
counselled that it is safe to do so within a few weeks of discharge
from hospital. Gradual resumption of former social activities should
be recommended during this time, as this has great psychological
benefit in demonstrating that he is capable of a normal and useful
life in the community. It should be stressed that some former
activities may not be suitable and that this is an opportunity to
cultivate new habits and interests.

The question of sedation and the use of tranquillizers is
important. The indications for their prescription and the possible
dangers of some of them are the same as in the acute phase. The
physician should emphasize the necessity for sleep and tranquillity
and should reassure the patient that the use of these drugs is for a
short time only. Their eventual withdrawal should be gradual.

Regular visits to the doctor and to members of the hospital
rehabilitation team are advisable to supervise the solution of
problems which have been identified earlier or to detect new problems
as they arise. Some patients may minimize sypmtoms and deny
emotional problems at follow up visits as they are afraid that they
may appear unmanly. Others may remain withdrawn or anxious even
though they may have coped satisfactorily during the acute phase.
A clue to the continued presence of anxiety or depression is
exaggerated compliance with medical advice and a certain satisfaction
at hearing the seriousness of his illness stressed by others.

Preparation for return to work signifies the end of
convalescence. The evidence is that this should not be unduly
delayed (about 6 - 8 weeks in the uncomplicated case). Contact
with the patient's employer beforehand about the individual's
ability to cope with his job will reduce uncertainty and help to
allay anxiety in both employer and employee.

Specialist rehabilitation services

The majority of patients, given this active approach from the
beginning of their illness will adapt satisfactorily to infarction.

The evidence is that the others will fail for a variety of different factors. Specialist rehabilitation services have been developed to improve outcome in these problem patients. Though the actual organi ation of these services varies from country to country and the particular emphasis in each centre may be different (physical retraining, psychological treatment, vocational guidance and training) the general principle of comprehensive rehabilitation applies to all. In these centres skilled rehabilitation teams can be concentrated so that a more detailed assessment of the patient's problems can be made and rehabilitation programmes tailored to the individual's needs instituted.

Group programmes. The psychological benefits of physical training are now known. There is subjective and objective evidence of improvement in physical fitness, anxiety and depression are lessened and the feeling of being treated as an invalid disappears. Group training permits communication with other individuals who have had similar experiences and face the same problems so that they tend to form a cohesive whole with support for individual members which no family,however understanding, can give. Group pressures also serve to cement resolutions about altering harmful habits and continuing with the physical training programme.

Psychological assessment and treatment. The assessment aims to evaluate the patient's potential capacity for work and perception of himself as an active member of the community. The methods include psychiatric interview and psychological testing of personality, emotional state and intelligence. Family members may be interviewed either at home or in the centre to estimate their personalities and attitudes to the patient's illness. Treatment will vary depending on the assessment but individual and group psychotherapy, with or without drugs to allay anxiety and to relieve depression, relaxation techniques, environmental and behaviour modifications are some of the measures already in use.

Vocational guidance. In patients whose physical capacity does not permit return to their previous employment, for whom no modification to their job is possible or who cannot return for legal reasons, the vocational expert must help them to find alternative employment. Evaluation of his previous work record, educational level, former training, his skills, interests, achievements and intelligence provides the necessary background information. As a result it is usually possible to specify a suitable type of job, taking into account his physical limitations and his special interests and abilities. If vocational retraining is going to be necessary, arrangements should be made to enter him for the appropriate course.

Inevitably, since these patients constitute a special "problem group" there will remain a number who by reason of physical disablement, age or severe defects of personality, remain

unemployable. It is usually possible to offer them some help,
such as sheltered workshop employment or guidance towards occupations
which they can do at home. An arrangement for domestic help may
permit the spouse to seek employment and in such a situation
psychological treatment of the patient may be necessary to help him
accept his more limited role.

Rehabilitation of patients after coronary bypass surgery

Since there is little evidence yet of the psychosocial factors
which retard or prevent successful rehabilitation in patients after
surgery, it is impossible to be dogmatic about treatment. Such
figures that are available at present suggest that their problems
are very similar to those in patients after a myocardial infarction,
so that it is reasonable to apply the same principles in treatment,
with special attention being directed to the possibility of
cerebral damage.

Post convalescent or maintenance phase

Return to work signifies the end of convalescence. It is
important to follow up the individual at least once to make sure
that he is coping both physically and psychologically. This is
especially important in those who have different or new jobs.
Rehabilitation after a myocardial infarction involves considerable
re-education and re-appraisal of the habits of a lifetime. A
continuing process of reinforcement may be necessary. For this
reason many rehabilitation centres offer continuing regular group
training. Some patients like to continue this indefinitely as they
find they have beneficial effects beyond maintenance of physical
fitness. Group pressures and friendly rivalry help to fortify such
people in their new healthy way of life, especially in relation to
eating habits, smoking and fitness. The recent growth of "coronary
clubs" and "heart clubs", a combination of social organizations and
disease-orientated clubs, in America set up and organized by former
patients is an example of this.

THE FUTURE

The last two decades have seen a revolution in the routine care
of the coronary patient. This is evidence in support of the
comprehensive approach in rehabilitation. But much remains to be
done.

Rehabilitation is still "patchy" and is not yet universally
seen as an integral part of patient care. There is need to
delineate much more clearly and objectively psychosocial outcome
both in terms of return to work and quality of life. Methods to
measure psychological and social factors in the coronary patient

are not yet satisfactory for routine clinical use. While various
psychological methods of treatment have been applied and have been
shown to benefit selected patients there is still an absence of
hard scientific data to prove their efficacy. We do not yet know
enough to delineate sub-groups which would benefit from a particular
therapy. There is little or no data comparing the results of
different types of rehabilitation programmes. The problem of
estimating the cost benefit of a rehabilitation programme as a
whole has barely been tackled, and the effects of individual
facets of a programme not yet considered.

References

1. F. M. Andrews and S. B. Witney. "Social indicators of well-
    being: Americans' perception of life quality." Plenum Press,
    New York, (1976).
2. F. J. Braceland. Psychiatric aspects. J. Rehab., 32: 53
    (1976).
3. N. H. Cassens and T. P. Hackett. Psychological rehabilitation
    of myocardial infarction patients in the acute phase. Heart
    and Lung, 2: 382, (1973).
4. R. B. Cattell. "The Specific Analysis of Personality".
    Penguin Books Ltd., Harmondsworth, (1965).
5. E. L. Cay, N. J. Vetter, A. Philip and P. Dugard. Psychological
    reactions to a coronary care unit. J. Psychosom Res., 16: 437
    (1972).
6. E. L. Cay, N. Vetter, A. Philip and P. Dugard. Psychological
    status during recovery from an acute heart attack. J. Psychosom
    Res., 16: 425 (1972).
7. E. L. Cay, N. Vetter, A. Philip and P. Dugard. Return to
    work after a heart attack. J. Psychosom Res., 17: 231 (1973).
8. E. L. Cay, N. J. Vetter and A. E. Philip. Practical aspects
    of cardiac rehabilitation: psychosocial factors. Giorn It
    Cardiol., 3: 646, (1973).
9. D. C. Coull, I. Crooks, I. Dingwall-Fordyce, A. M. Scott and
    M. D. Weir. Amitryptyline and cardiac disease: risk of
    sudden death identified by monitoring system. Lancet, 2: 590
    (1970).
10. M. Dobson, A. E. Tattersfield, M. M. Adler and M. W. McNicol.
    Attitudes and long term adjustment of patients surviving
    cardiac arrest. Br. Med. J., 3: 207 (1971).
11. J. Dominian and M. Dobson. Study of patients' psychological
    attitudes to a coronary care unit. Brit Med J., 4: 795
    (1979).
12. R. G. Druss and D. S. Kornfeld. Survivors of cardiac
    arrest: psychiatric study JAMA, 201: 291 (1967).
13. E. F. Dunbar. "Psychosomatic Diagnosis". Paul P. Hoeber,
    New York (1943).

14. S. H. Fisher Mechanism of denial in physical disability.
    Arch Neurol Psychiat., 80: 782 (1958).
15. A. H. Goble, G. H. Adey and J. F. Bullen. Rehabilitation of
    the cardiac patient. Med. J. Aust., 2: 975 (1963).
16. D. P. Goldberg and B. Blackwell. Psychiatric illness in
    general practice: a detailed study using a new method of
    case identification. Brit Med J., 2: 439 (1970).
17. B. M. Groden and R. I.P. Brown. Differential psychological
    effects of early and late mobilization after myocardial
    infarction. Scand J Rehab Med., 2: 60 (1970).
18. T. P. Hackett, N. H. Cassens and H. A. Wishnie. Detection and
    treatment of anxiety in the coronary care unit. Am Heart J.
    78: 727 (1969).
19. T. P. Hackett and N. H. Cassens. Development of a quantitive
    rating scale to assess denial. J Psychosom Res., 18: 93
    (1974).
20. T. P. Hackett. "Coronary Care: Patient Psychology".
    American Heart Association, Inc. (1975).
21. T. P. Hackett. The use of groups in the rehabilitation of
    the post-coronary patient. p. 120. In: "Advances in
    Cardiology: Cardiac Rehabilitation". K. König and H. Denolin,
    ed., Karger, Basel, (1978).
22. H. Hellerstein and A. Ford. Rehabilitation of the cardiac
    patient. JAMA 164: 225 (1957).
23. H. Hellerstein et al. Active physical conditioning of
    coronary patients. Circulation, 32: 100 (1965).
24. H. Hellerstein and E. H. Friedman. Sexual activity and the
    post-coronary patient. Arch Int Med., 125: 987 (1970).
25. D. Jenkins. "Toward a redefinition of the coronary-prone
    behaviour pattern: Inferences from test items which predict
    future coronary disease." Lecture at the Annual Meeting of
    the American Psychosomatic Society, Philadelphia (1974).
26. J. J. Kellermann. "The physical evaluation and rehabilitation
    of patients with coronary heart disease." In: Proceedings
    of the First International Biennial Conference on Cardiac
    Rehabilitation, Dubrovnik Plavsic and Gertler, ed., (1970).
27. J. Kellermann. "Rehabilitation of coronary patients". Final
    report, 1970.
28. "Stress and Distress in Response to Psychosocial Stimuli",
    Almqvist and Wiksell, L. Levi, ed., Stockholm, (1972).
29. S. A. Levine and B. Lown. Armchair treatment of acute
    coronary thrombosis. JAMA 148: 1365 (1952).
30. "Long-Term Effects of Cornary Bypass Surgery". Report of a
    Working Group, The Hague, WHO, Regional Office for Europe,
    Copenhagen, (1977).
31. A. J. Mandel. The psychological management of coronary
    patients, GP., 27: 82 (1963).
32. R. Mayou, A. Foster and B. Williamson. The psychological
    and social effects of myocardial infarction on wives.
    Brit Med J., 1: 699-701 (1978).

33. "Myocardial Infarction: How to prevent. How to Rehabilitate", Symposium of the Scientific Council on Rehabilitation, International Society of Cardiology, Vienna, T. Semple et al ed., Boehringer Mannheim, (1973).

34. R. Nagle, R. Gangola and I. Picton-Robertson. Factors influencing return to work after myocardial infarction, Lancet, 11 : 454 (1971).

35. J. Naughton et al. Rehabilitation for patients after myocardial infarction. Southern Med Bill, 55: 29 (1967).

36. J. P. Naughton and H. K. Hellerstein. "Exercise Testing and Exercise Training in Coronary Heart Disease". Academic Press, New York, (1971).

37. Short-term fluctuations in anxiety in patients with myocardial infarction. A. E. Philip, E. L. Cay, N. J. Vetter and N. A. Stuckey. J. Psychosom Res., (in press).

38. "Psychological Approach to the Rehabilitation of Coronary Patients". Symposium of the Scientific Council on Rehabilitation International Society of Cardiology, Höhenried V. Stocksmeier, ed., Springer-Verlag, Berlin (1976).

39. "Psychological Aspects of the Rehabilitation of Cardiovascular Patients." Report of a Working Group, Warsaw WHO, Regional Office for Europe, Copenhagen, (1969).

40. "Psychological Problems in Cardiac Rehabilitation". Symposium of the Scientific Council on Rehabilitation International Society of Cardiology, Zurich, K. König and H. Denolin, ed., Gödecke A. G, (1976).

41. Proceedings of a symposium, Council on Rehabilitation, International Society of Cardiology, Cambridge, Scand J Rehab Med., 2 (1970).

42. C. J. Rabiner and A. E. Willner. Psychopathology observed on follow-up after cornary bypass surgery. J Nerv Ment Dis., 163: 295 (1976).

43. R. H. Rahe, M. Romo, L. Bennett and Siltanen. Recent life changes, myocardial infarction and abrupt coronary death. Arch Int Med., 133: 221 (1974).

44. W. R. Rogers. Evaluation of the cardiac patients for empolyment, J Occup Med., 4: 73 (1962).

45. D. M. Rumbaugh. Prediction of work potential in heart patients through the use of the cardiac adjustment scale. J Consul Psychol., 29: 597 (1964).

46. H. D. Ruskin et al. MMPI: comparison between patients with coronary heart disease and their spouses together with other demographic data, Scand J Rehab Med., 2: 99 (1970.

47. I. H. and R. B. Cattell. Handbook for IPAT 8-parallel Form Anxiety Battery Champaign IPAT, (1960).

48. E. Schiller and F. Baker. Return to work after a myocardial infarction: evaluation of planned rehabilitation and of a predictive rating scale. Med J Aust., 1: 859-862 (1976).

49. H. Selye and E. Bajusz. Conditioning by corticoids for the production of cardiac lesions with noradrenalin, <u>Acta. Endocrinol</u>, 30: 183 (1959).
50. J. Singh, S. Singh, S. Singh, A. Singh and R. P. Malhotra. Sex life and psychiatric problems after myocardial infarction, <u>J Assn Physicians India</u>, 18: 503 (1970).
51. "Some factors in the work adjustment of cardiac patients". Alameda County Heart Assoc., Alameda, California, (1962).
52. C. D. Spielberger, R. L. Gorsuch and R. Lushens, STAI Manual, Palo Alto, California, Consulting Psychologists Press, (1970).
53. M. J. Stern, L. Pascale and J. B. McLoone. Psychosocial adaptation following an acute myocardial infarction. <u>J. Chron Dis</u>., 29: 513 (1976).
54. T. Theorell and R. H. Rahe. Behaviour and life satisfaction: characteristics of Swedish subjects with myocardial infarction <u>J Chron Dis</u>., 25: 139 (1972).
55. W. B. Tuttle and W. L. Cook. Sexual behaviour in post-myocardial infarction patients. <u>Am J Cardiol</u>., 13: 140 (1964).
56. M. Ueno. The so-called coition death. <u>Jap J of Legal Med</u>., 17: 333 (1963).
57. N. N. Wagner. Sexual adjustment of cardiac patients. <u>Brit J of Sexual</u> Med., 1: 17 (1974).
58. P. A. Whitehouse. Some psychological factors that influence the rehabilitation of the cardiac. <u>J Rehab</u>., 4: 32 (1960).
59. A. Wynn. Unwarranted emotional distress in men with ischemic heart disease. <u>Med J Aust</u>., 2: 847 (1967).
60. L. R. Zohman and J. S. Tobis. "Cardiac Rehabilitation". Grune and Stratton, New York, (1970).

PLANNING OF COMPREHENSIVE REHABILITATION ON THE BASIS OF

EXERCISE TESTING AFTER MYOCARDIAL INFARCTION

E. Kentala

Kiljava Hospital

Finland

INTRODUCTION

The range of physical working capacity (PWC) after myocardial
infarction is wide (Fig.1) (9), and therefore, exercise testing
is essential for realistic rehabilitation plans. Physical
training has been one promising method of improving PWC when
there is a gap between physical fitness and the demands of the
work. In two controlled Finnish studies, however, intervention
with physical training alone did not induce any significant
improvement in return to work, or in mortality. In our
feasibility study with consecutive postinfarction men (Fig.1) (9)
the effect of one year's physical activity programme was not
very protracted (Fig. 2). Mortality was similar and return to
work tended to be better in the reference group (Fig. 3) when
the basic treatment, including exercise tests and follow-up
examinations, was the same in both groups. So, psychosocial
and local factors seems to be much more important in return
to work than physical fitness. In similar Finnish study on
physical training, results regarding return to work and mortality
were the same , although there was a slight trend towards
lower mortality in the training group (17). In the recent
comprehensive rehabilitation and secondary prevention study
co-ordinated by WHO, however, more favourable results were achieved
(7). The incidence of sudden death in men during the first,
vulnerable year after myocardial infarction was particularly
reduced. In this study, all possible secondary prevention
measures, in addition to physical training programme, were
included and the patients of the reference group were first
examined one year after infarction by the members of the research
team; this constitutes an important difference compared to the

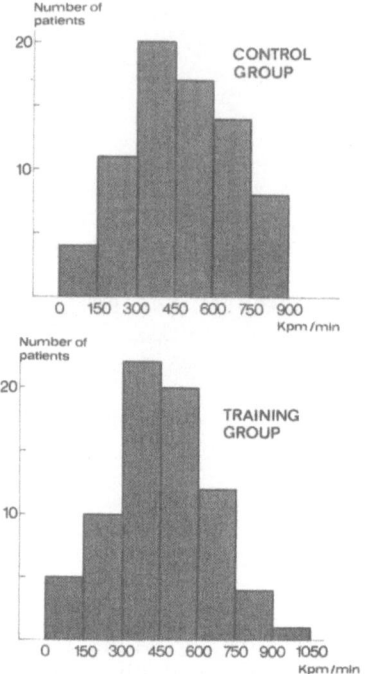

Fig. 1. Distribution of physical working capacity 6-8 weeks
         after acute myocardial infarction in connection with a
         rehabilitation study (9).

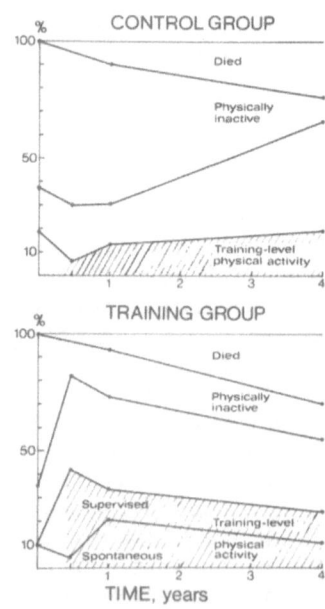

Fig. 2. Physical activity during the follow-up period in the
         training group and in the control group.

aforementioned studies. Therefore, at this stage, it is difficult
to say by which means the favourable result was achieved. Was it
physical training, or better nutrition education and lower serum
cholesterol, better medication and stricter blood pressure control
or simply closer physician-patient relationship?

PROGNOSTIC ASPECTS

    To answer the question posed at the end of the preceding chapter,
prognostic aspects of myocardial infarction must be discussed.
The possibility of changing of those factors which have the greatest
prognostic significance in this phase of ischaemic heart disease
would, of course, lead to the most favourable results in
comprehensive rehabilitation.

    In our series, 51 of 158 patients died from coronary heart
disease during the 6 years follow-up period. Sudden death
(within 1 hour) was more common during the last trimester of the
follow-up period (Fig. 4). Stepwise multiple discriminant analysis
with the 18 best, simple and non-invasive variables was used to
delineate the most important prognostic factors (Fig. 5) (13). In
the 2-year prognosis, low systolic blood pressure at maximal work
load was the most unfavourable finding. These patients seemed to
have the poorest left ventricular function, which was incapable
of coping with increased afterload during exercise. In 4 and
6-year cumulative analyses, however, accentuated P-terminal
force of resting ECG, depicting increased pre-load (a slighter
functional disturbance of the left ventricle) had the greatest
discriminatory power. In the second discriminant analysis, these
six best variables were combined with some classical risk factors
of coronary heart disease (Fig. 6). Smoking was the most important
traditional risk factor, but was exceeded greatly by variables
associated with poor left ventricular function

Sudden or Non-Sudden Death

    During the last trimester of the follow-up period, when sudden
death was most common, the discriminatory power of post-exercise
T-wave changes was enhanced (Fig. 5). This is not surprising
because the inhomogeneity of ventricular repolarization is a factor
in both T-wave-form and arrhythmia vulnerability (4). Prolongation of
the QT interval has also been suggested as one ECG manifestation
of increased disparity of ventricular refractory periods. Therefore,
QT times were also checked in this series. There was no difference
in rate-corrected QT times in resting supine measurements. During
somatomotor activation, however, when the patient has mounted a
bicycle for exercise testing, QT_c time appeared to be significantly
longer in patients with subsequent sudden death (Fig. 7) (11).

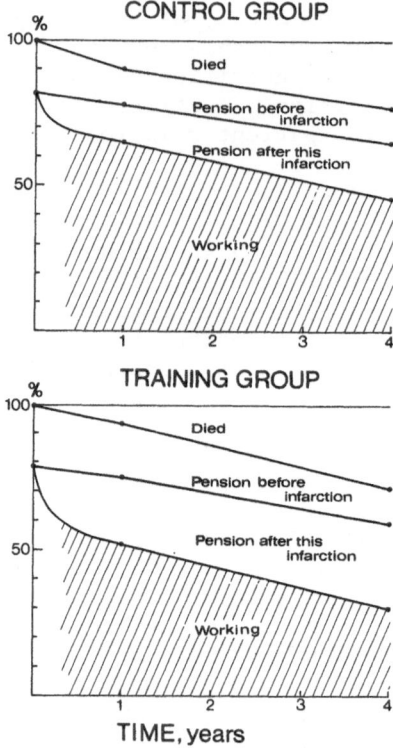

Fig. 3. Mortality and return to work in the study population
        with 158 patients.

This reaction might be very similar with fight or flight reaction,
which the patient often meets in daily life.

     On the other hand, R-wave amplitude at the beginning of
exercise, when there is normally an overshoot of sympathetic tone,
was lower in the non-sudden death group (Fig.8) (12). It is tempting
to explain this by saying that the left ventricular response to
exercise is disturbed because of impaired autonomic innervation.
The heart in the non-sudden death group might react to exercise in
a way similar to a denervated heart by increasing the stroke volume
in accordance with the Frank-Starling mechanism (8) rather than by
adrenergic response and higher R-wave amplitude, as in the other
groups. In the sudden death group the possible denervation process
or myocardial catecholamine depletion might not be so diffuse and
there are obviously also highly activa areas inducing imbalance in
the cardiac sympathetic neuronal stimulation, which could lead to
prolongation of the QT interval.

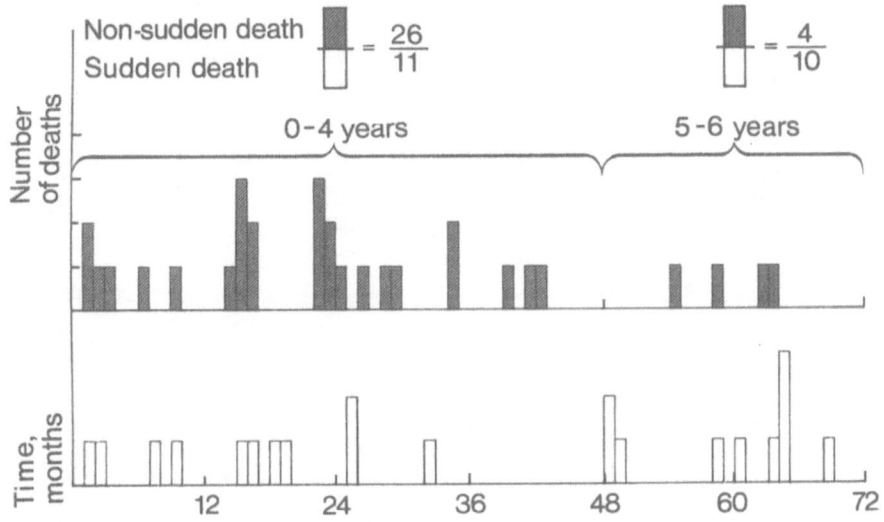

Fig. 4. Sudden and non-sudden deaths during a 6-year follow-up period (13).

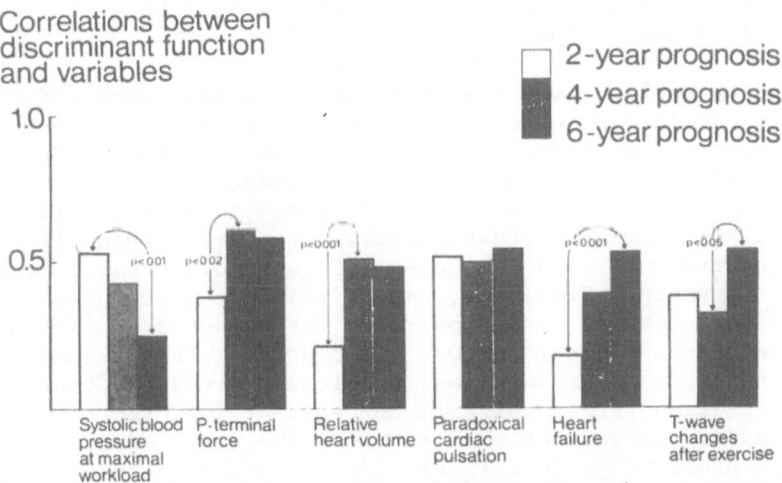

Fig. 5. Correlations between discriminant function and some of the most important clinical variables in stepwise multiple discriminant analysis made on the basis of 2, 4 and 6-year cumulative mortality with the same pattern of 18 selected variables (13).

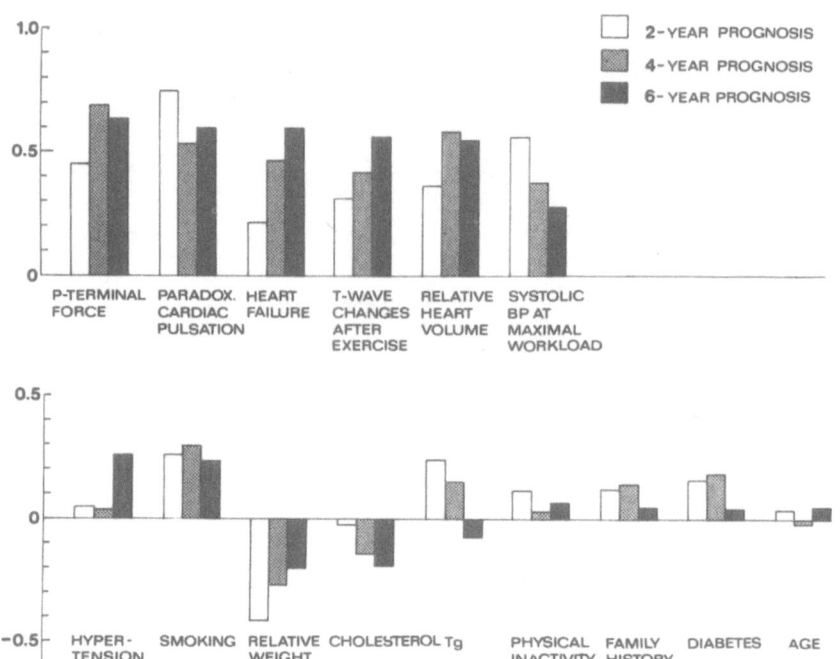

Fig. 6.   The six best prognostic variables associated with poor
          left ventricular function compared by stepwise multiple
          discriminant analysis with some traditional risk factors
          of coronary heart disease. Correlations between
          discriminant function and variables.

     Heart rate-blood pressure products at maximal workload were,
by chance, similar in sudden and in non-sudden death groups.
In the sudden death group, however, heart rate tended to be higher
and blood pressure lower than in the non-sudden death group (Fig.9),
which fits with the hypothesis that response to exercise is
different. ST segment depression during exercise, which is
compatible with multivessel disease (19),was more usual in the
sudden death group. Similarly, P-terminal force, measured 5
minutes after exercise in supine rest, was accentuated in the
sudden death group (Fig.10) (10). It might be, that these
patients had more severe proximal critical lesions and therefore
a slow relaxation rate in significant part of left ventricular wall
and delayed recovery after exercise. On the other hand, the heart
rate-blood pressure product is already decreased in this phase, and
mechanisms other than increased oxygen demand, e.g. coronary artery
spasm, might be responsible for delayed recovery of left ventricular
function. This possibility fits with the fact that coronary artery
spasm is often preceeded by QT_c interval prolongation (18).

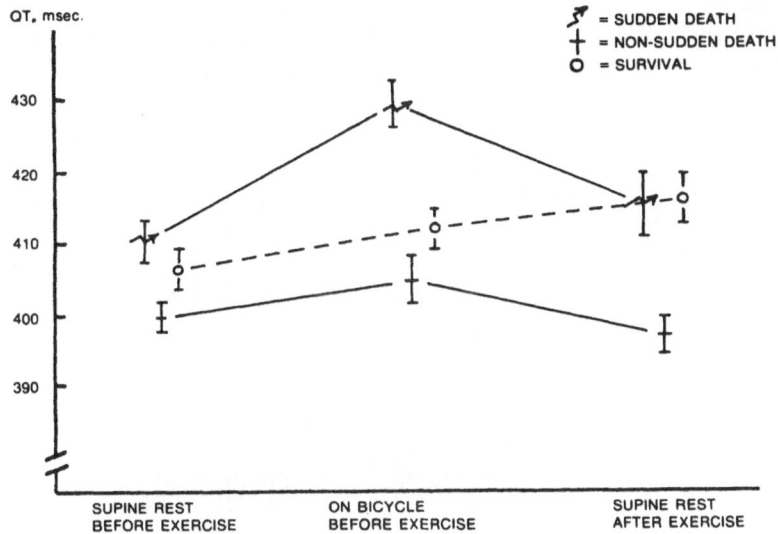

Fig. 7. Mean and S.E. values of corrected QT time (QT$_c$) in patients with previous acute myocardial infarction (11).

Individual Plans for Rehabilitation

This prognostic and haemodynamic mosaicism must be taken into account when planning comprehensive rehabilitation and rehabilitation studies.

Theoretically, three main crude haemodynamic groups may be delineated in postinfarction patients (Fig. 11). In the best group, pump function and perfusion are quite intact and the heart can normally increase ejection fraction by adrenergic mechanisms during exercise. PWC is good, no ST segment depression is seen, and there is normal variation of R-wave amplitude during exercise. The prognosis is good and there is sufficient time for secondary preventive measures..

In the second group, the ejection fraction at rest and at the beginning of exercise is good but exercise later reveals poor pump function due mainly to poor myocardial perfusion. Angina pectoris, ST segment depression compatible with multivessel disease and terminal drop in systolic blood pressure during exercise

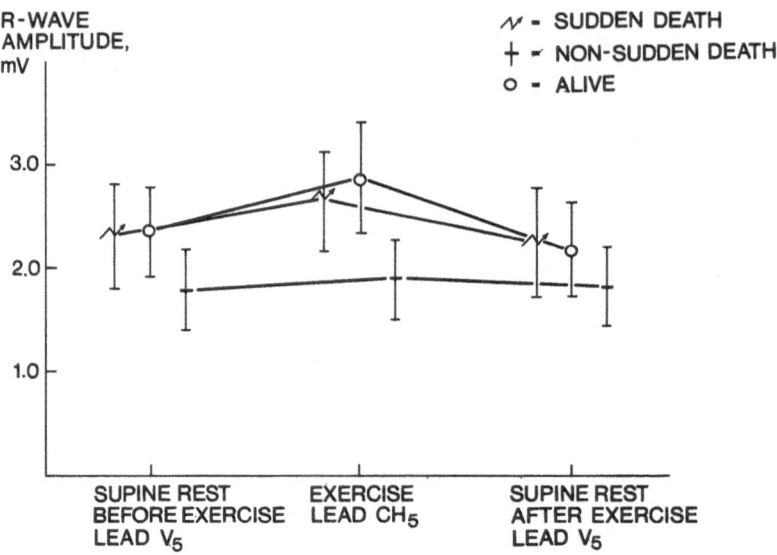

Fig. 8. Mean and S.D. values of R-wave amplitudes in connection
         with postinfarction exercise testing.

are seen. After exercise ischaemic functional disturbance
of the left ventricle usually disappears when the heart rate-blood
pressure product decreases. In patients who can be expected to die
suddenly, however, other factors, such as coronary artery spasm,
complicate recovery. This might be depicted by accentuation of
P-terminal force after exercise despite the decreasing oxygen
demands of the left ventricule.

     In the third group with poorest prognosis, left ventricular
ejection fraction is already poor at rest. These patients can not
normally increase blood pressure during exercise. PWC and heart
rate-blood pressure product are low, and R wave amplitude changes
are minimal. Instead of ST segment depression, no change or ST
segment elevation, which has been shown to be associated with
common left ventricular aneurysms in this group (19), are seen.

     In the first group prognosis is so good that it takes many
years to see possible improvement by secondary prevention measures
and physical training.

     The most intensive and versatile rehabilitation measures
are needed in the second group where cardiac muscle is not yet
too seriously damaged. In debilitating angina pectoris with
multivessel disease, a coronary-artery bypass operation to enhance

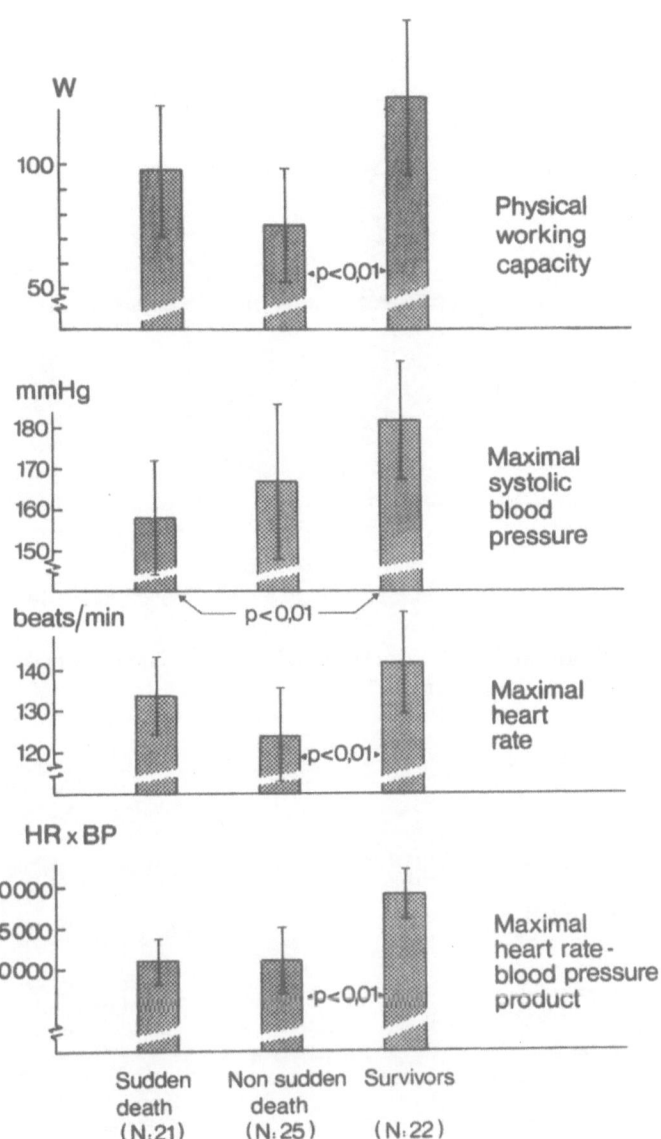

Fig. 9. Mean and S.D. values of PWC, heart rate and systolic
         blood pressure at maximal physical exertion in patients
         with different fates during the subsequent 6-year
         follow-up period.

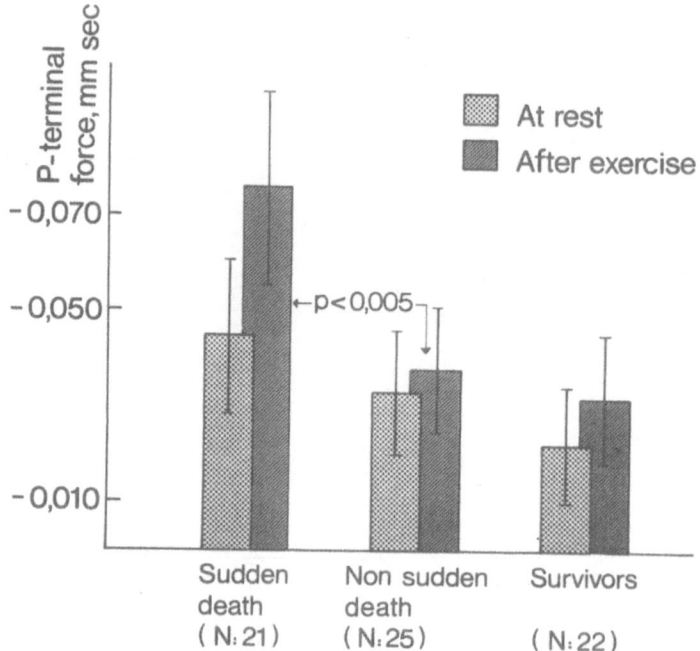

Fig. 10.   Mean and S.D. values of P-terminal force at rest and
            after exercise.

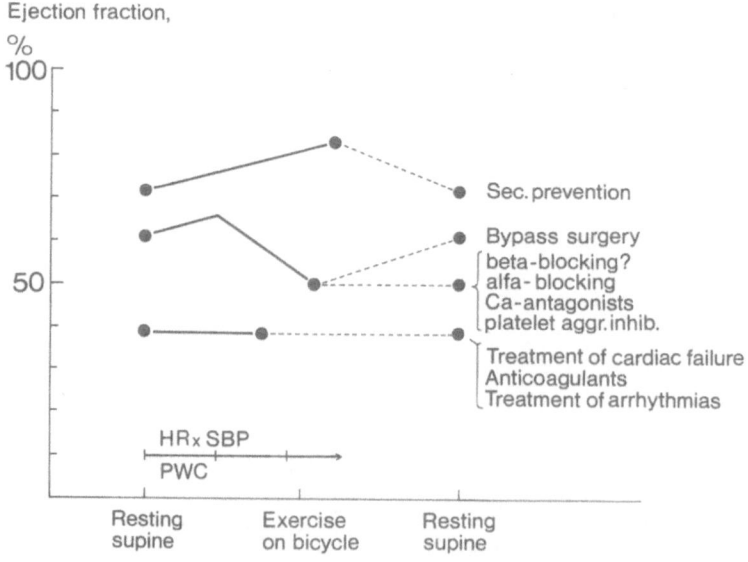

Fig. 11.   Theoretical grouping of postinfarction patients for plan-
            ning of comprehensive rehabilitation (details in test).

the myocardial oxygen supply seems justified. With regard to drug therapy, beta-adrenergic blockade is usually beneficial in patients with typical angina pectoris by decreasing myocardial oxygen demands. Reduction in the incidence of sudden death by beta-blocking drugs has also been reported (20). The problem is when and to what extent coronary artery spasm is involved in etiology of sudden death. A heavy parasympathomimetic braking action of the heart appears during supine rest after exercise testing when metabolic coronary vasodilatation is disappearing. Parasympathetic stimulation can also indirectly activate the sympathetic nerves leading to alpha-adrenergic vasoconstriction of the coronary arteries (6) and reveal patients prone to coronary artery spasm. Typical ST segment elevation, however, is a rare finding in coronary patients and perhaps other signs of functional disturbance of the left ventricle caused by coronary artery spasm should be investigated. Stimulation of beta-2 receptors, which induces vasodiliatation in coronary arteries, is blocked by non-selective beta-blocking drugs. Their use may actually be harmful if ischaemia is due to reduced oxygen supply secondary to coronary spasm (3). On the other hand, propranolol reduces platelet aggregation during pacing in the coronary circulation of patients with coronary artery disease (15). In patients with multivessel disease and good pump function, platelet damage and aggregation might be significant in coronary circulation during exercise, too. Production and release of thromboxane A_2 may also promote coronary artery spasm during the postexercise period, and it is not counteracted by prostacyclin I_2 because of endothelial damage of the coronary arteries. This could explain some promising results in secondary prevention with platelet aggregation inhibitors (1). The role of alpha-blocking drugs and Ca-antagonists in secondary prevention of coronary heart disease is not yet clear.

Because the main problem in this group is poor perfusion, it can hardly be solved by physical training. The post-training increase in exercise tolerance of patients with angina pectoris does not depend on an augmented myocardial oxygen supply, but is related to a reduction in coronary flow requirements for a given absolute work load (5,16). Subendocardial oxygen supply might be better in relation to total myocardial oxygen demands after a training period (2) but the effect on morbidity and mortality had not yet been proved.

In the third group, poor pump function due to loss of viable muscle is the main problem. Physical training cannot improve left ventricular function, as shown by Letac and Nolewajka (14,16). Achievement of peripheral training effect is also quite impossible, because low cardiac output already forces peripheral muscles to increase their oxygen extraction capacity. Therefore, treatment of cardiac failure, prevention of thromboembolic complications and

treatment and prevention of arrhythmias associated with ventricular
aneurysms, which are common in this group, are the main tasks for
the attending physician.

However, the fact that arrhythmia leading to sudden death
comes only once means that identification and treatment of the
preceeding disturbance to the cardiac haemodynamics, platelet
function or autonomic innervation might be more rewarding than
treatment of arrhythmias. Knowing the central role of autonomic
nervous system in coronary heart disease, the importance of
psychological factors and close patient-physician relationship can
not be overestimated in comprehensive rehabilitation.

References

1. The Anturane reinfarction trial research group: Sulfinpyrazone
    in the prevention of cardiac death after myocardial infarction
    N. Engl. J. Med. 298:289 (1978).
2. R. J. Barnard, R. Mac Alpin, A. A. Kattus, G. D. Buckberg,
    Effect of training on myocardial oxygen supply/demand balance.
    Circ. 56:281 (1977).
3. E. Braunwald, Coronary spasm and acute myocardial infarction -
    new possibility for treatment and prevention. N. Engl. J.
    Med. 299:1301 (1978).
4. M. J. Burgess, Relation of ventricular repolarization to
    electrocardiographic T wave-form and arrhythmia vulnerability.
    AM. J. Physiol. 236:H391 (1979).
5. R. J. Ferguson, P. Côté, P. Gauthier, M. G. Bourassa, Changes in
    exercise coronary sinus blood flow with training in patients
    with angina pectoris, Circ. 58:41 (1978).
6. L. D. Hillis, E. Braunwald, Coronary artery spasm, N.Engl.
    J. Med. 299:695 (1978).
7. V. Kallio, H. Hämäläinen, J. Hakkila, O. Luurila, Reduction of
    sudden deaths after a multifactorial intervention programme
    in patients after acute myocardial infarction. To be published.
8. K. M. Kent, T. Cooper, The denervated heart. A model for
    studying autonomic control of the heart, N. Engl. J. Med.
    291:1017 (1974).
9. E. Kentala, Physical fitness and feasibility of physical
    rehabilitation after myocardial infarction in men of working
    age, Ann Clin. Res. 4, Suppl. 9 (1972).
10. E. Kentala, Discrimination between subsequent sudden and non-
    sudden death by postinfarction exercise testing. Scand. J.
    Rehab. Med. 8:73 (1976).
11. E. Kentala, U.K. Repo, QT-interval prolongation during
    somatomotor activation as predictor of sudden death after
    myocardial infarction, Ann Clin. Res. 11:42 (1979).
12. E. Kentala, U. K. Repo, Low exercise R wave amplitude after
    myocardial infarction predicting subsequent non-sudden
    death, to be published.

13. E. Kentala, S. Sarna, Sudden death and factors related to long-term prognosis following acute myocardial infarction, Scand. J. Rehab. Med. 8:27 (1976).

14. B. Letac, A. Cribbier, J. F. Desplanches, A study of left ventricular function in coronary patients before and after physical training, Circ. 56:375 (1977).

15. J. Mehta, P. Mehta, C. J. Pepine, Platelet aggregation in aortic and coronary venous blood in patients with and without coronary disease, 3. Role of tachycardia stress and propranolol, Circ. 58:881 (1978).

16. A. J. Nolewajka, W. J. Kostuk. P. A. Rechnitzer, D. A. Cunningham, Exercise and human collateralization: An angiographic and scintigroaphic assessment, Circ.60:114 (1979).

17. I. Palatsi, Feasibility of physical training after myocardial infarction and its effect on return to work, morbidity and mortality, Acta Med. Scand. Suppl. 599, (1976).

18. D. R. Ricci, A. E. Orlick, R. P. Cipriano, D.F. Guthaner, D.C. Harrison, Altered adrenergic activity in coronary arterial spasm, Insight into mechanism based on study of coronary hemodynamics and the electrocardiogram, Am. J. Cardiol. 43:1073 (1979).

19. D. A. Weiner, C. McCabe, M. D. Klein, T. J. Ryan, ST segment changes post-infarction: Predictive value for multivessel coronary disease and left ventricular aneurysm, Circ. 58:887(1978).

20. C. Wilhelmsson, A. Vedin, L. Wilhelmsen, G. Tibblin, L. Werkö: Reduction of sudden deaths after myocardial infarction by treatment with alprenolol, Lancet 2:1157 (1974).

THE TRAINING EFFECT IN SHORT TERM REHABILITATION

K. König

Herz-Kreislauf-Klinik
Waldkirch
Federal Republic of Germany

In my short report I would like to talk about the results of 1200 patients after myocardial infarction; these patients underwent a fully controlled exercise program during so-called institutional rehabilitation in our clinic. The duration of the program was from 4 to 6 weeks. As you know, the development of rehabilitation after myocardial infarction in specially equipped rehabilitation centers is rather advanced in the Federal Republic of Germany. We believe, that with this form of so-called comprehensive rehabilitation, we get very good results in a very short time. When talking about rehabilitation in special centers, we must differentiate between:

1. Early rehabilitation, immediately following discharge from the hospital according to Phase II of WHO-Classification and

2. Repeated Rehabilitation, months or years after the infarction during Phase III.

First some short remarks concerning the applied methods. The initial and final examinations are made up of: Heart Volume, determined by X-Ray; Ergometric Tests in supine position. The parameter for the maximal working capacity is the maximal oxygen pulse.

The weekly rehabilitation program contains the following activities: When no counterindication is given, the patients perform 15 minutes of daily exercise on the ergometer. During the first three months after the infarction, the exercise intensity is increased according to the patient's working tolerance. In

the period 3 months after infarction, the patient exercises with
70 per cent of his maximal working capacity. Other activities
are: Gymnastics, walking at different distances, swimming, and
various froms of hydrotherapy.

In the following Figures I would like to demonstrate some
results regarding the effect of exercise on heart rate, heart
rate - blood pressure product, and maximal working capacity.

First the heart rate; bradycardia resulting from physical
training has been shown in numerous studies to be similar in
healthy individuals as in coronary patients.

The special significance of lowering the pulse frequency
by physical training lies, especially for coronary patients in
the decrease of the oxygen need for the heart muscle. The heart,
therefore, needs as result of the decrease of the heart frequency
by training for a given task less oxygen than before the onset
of training.

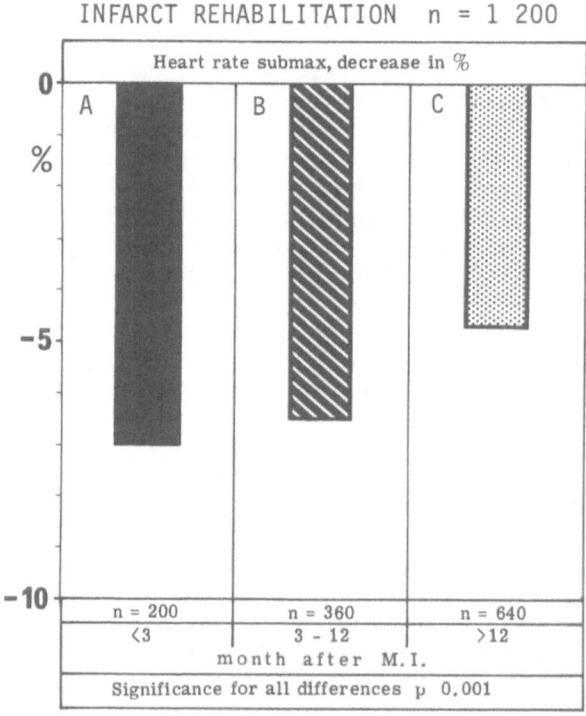

Figure 1.

In this Figure the entire collective was divided into
three groups. In Group A the infarction had occurred less than
3 months before. In Group B it had occurred between 3 and 12
months before, and in Group C the time between infarction and
rehabilitation was over 12 months. The latter cases involved
repeated treatment in the rehabilitation center. During the
first 3 months after myocardial infarction, it means in Group
A the reduction in heart rate is the greatest with minus 7%.
This corresponds to the still very retarded work efficiency of
a heart damaged by infarction. As the time since the infarction
increases, the percentage reduction in heart rate diminished to
minus 4.7%. For all 3 Groups, however, the extent of the
reduction in heart rate is statistically highly significant.

The diminution of the heart work is not only a result of
bradycardia, but results also from a decrease in the cardiac
pressure work, which is indicated by the decrease in the
peripheral blood-pressure. In our study we found highly significant
reductions in the systolic blood-pressure at rest and for identical
submaximal work loads. Better than the heart rate or the blood
pressure alone as an indicator for the efficiency of heart
function is the combined product of both factors. This product of

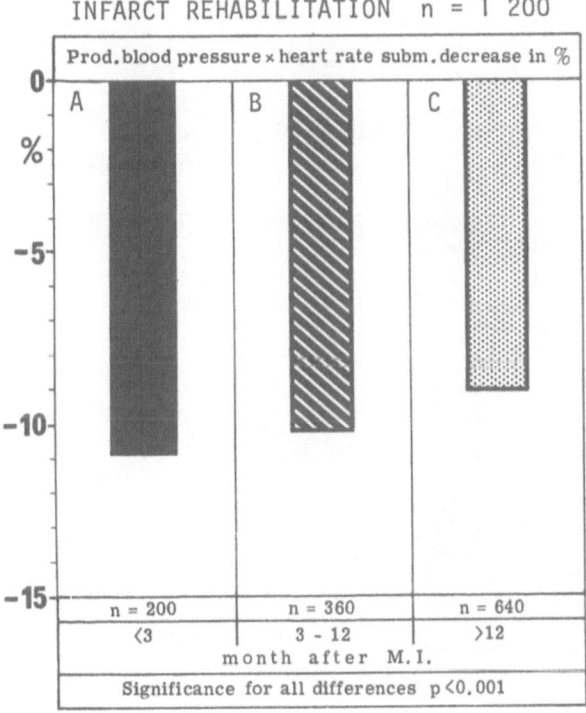

Figure 2.

the heart rate and the blood-pressure is proportional to the
myocardial oxygen consumption; as Figure 2 shows, the decrease
of the blood-pressure - pulse product during sub-maximal load
was highly significant in all Groups. The amount was the highest
in Group A at minus 10.8% and reduced itself to minus 9% in
Group C.

What about the working capacity? At the end of the 4 to 6
week rehabilitation period, the maximal oxygen pulse increased
by pulse 38% in Group A. This remarkable increase in performance
at the beginning of Phase II is understandable, since infarction
had occurred only a relatively short time ago. Therefore, these
patients had a very low capacity at the beginning of the
exercise therapy. As expected, the rates of increase were only
14 to 10 percent respectively in the later stage of rehabilitation.
These performance increases are statistically of high significance.

A very interesting result was obtained by measuring the
X-Ray determined heart volume before and after the 4 to 6 week
rehabilitation period. This can be seen in the Figure 4.
In all 3 Groups there were highly significant reductions in
heart size. Again the most pronounced reduction was found in
the patients of Group A at the beginning of Phase II.

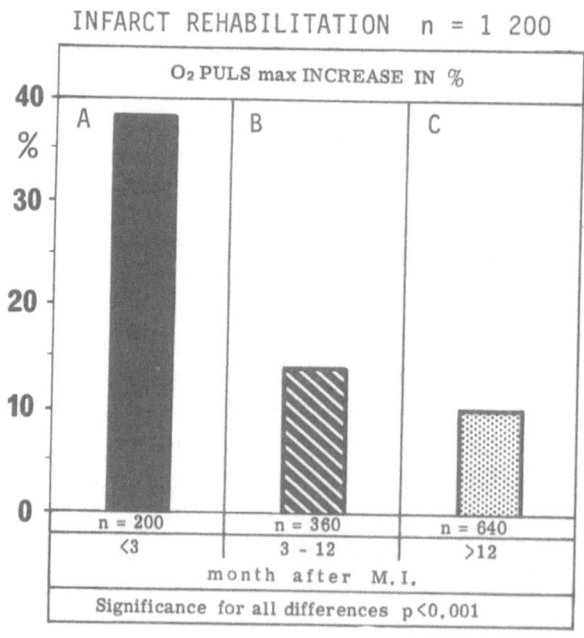

Figure 3.

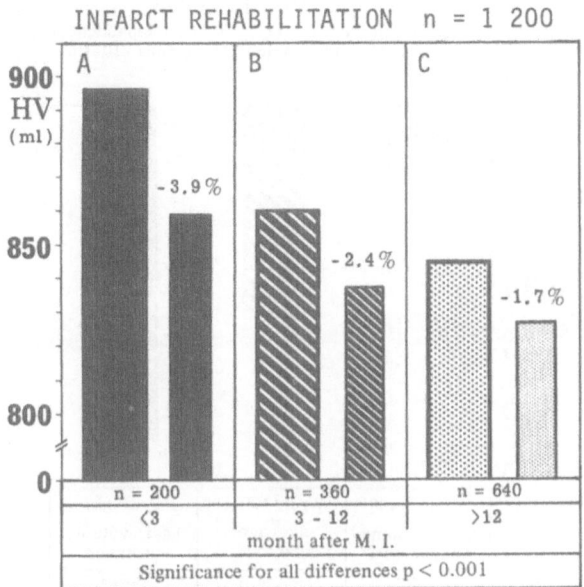

Figure 4.

One argument explaining this highly significant reduction
in heart size is, that in the acute infarction phase a
compensatory enlargement of the heart occurs in the sense of the
Frank-Starling mechanism, depending on the size of the scar and
the loss of contractile substance. In this case, the enlargement
can be connected to a reduction of contractility and an increase
of ventricular filling pressure. So, reduction in size of
the heart means, that the loss of contraction caused by the scar
has been compensated by the remaining healthy myocardium.

The connection between size of the heart on one hand and
the reduced muscle contractility as result of the infarct on the
other hand is supported by the fact, that the initial heart
volume during the first months following infarct was the largest
in Group A and is pronounced smaller in Groups B and C where the
infarct had occurred earlier. In this context it becomes clear,
why the percentage-wise decrease rates in the early stage after
the infarct are larger than during later phases.

When during exercise therapy an enlargement of the heart
volume is found, it indicates negative development. The heart
enlargement is proof, that the heart has been overloaded by
physical training. In such cases, physical activity must be
reduced for a certain time. Such an enlargement of the heart is
also a sign, that Digitalization is urgently needed.

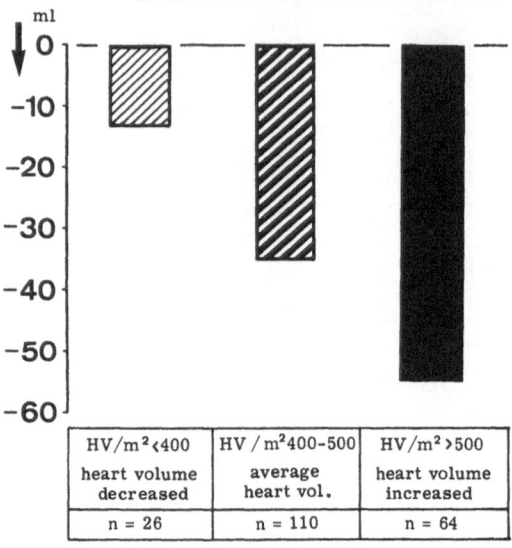

INFARCT REHABILITATION
Decreased heart volume after rehabilitation dependent on
initial heart volume before rehabilitation

HV/m²<400 heart volume decreased	HV/m²400-500 average heart vol.	HV/m²>500 heart volume increased
n = 26	n = 110	n = 64

Figure 5.

The following Figure analyses the question, whether the
degree of heart volume decrease depends on the initial heart
volume at the onset of rehabilitation. It shows indeed, that
in small hearts, with a heart volume per body surface under 400,
only minor heart volume decrease is found after 4 to 6 weeks.
When the heart volume is in the upper normal range, the decrease
is much more pronounced. The largest volume decreases are
found, as expected, in pathologically enlarged hearts.

In healthy individuals there exists, as well known, a close
correlation between the size of the heart and the performance
capacity, that means, the larger the heart, the better the
performance. The question arises, whether the degree of
performance improvement after training depends on the size of
the initial heart volume also for infarct patients.

On Figure 6 a division into normal and enlarged hearts
was made on the abscissa. The Figure shows, that the improvement
of performance of a small heart is the greatest. With larger
heart volumina the performance improvement is progressingly
decreasing. As an explanation for this phenomena we again
have to refer to the above made hypothesis. It means, that a
small heart may be an expression of a small infarction or a
good compensation of the infarct scar by the remaining healthy
myocardium. Such hearts have more favourable contractile reserves.

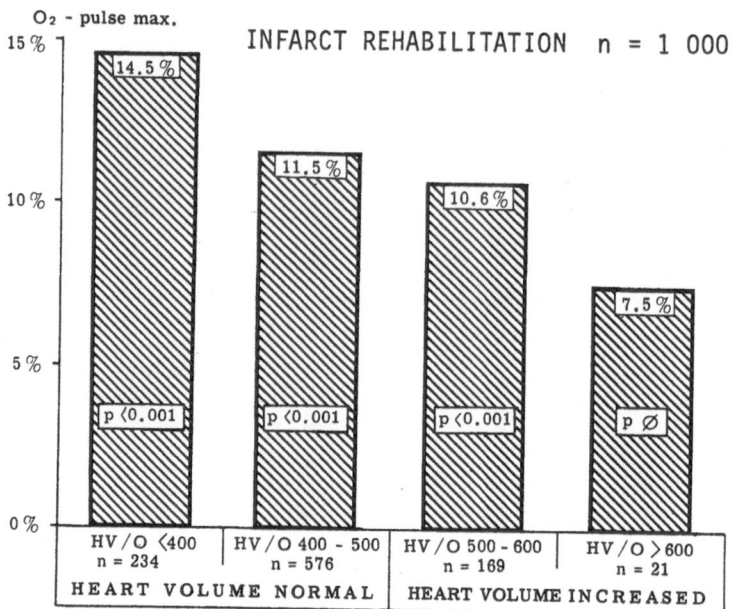

Increase of max.O_2 - pulse after rehabilitation dependent
on initial heart volume before rehabilitation

Figure 6.

Exercise therapy will, for this reason, result in the best
performance of these hearts. Large hearts, on the other hand,
may be connected with large infarcts, respectively poorly
compensated infarct scars, which led to dilatation of the heart.
Such hearts will have relatively few contractile reserves. Exercise
therapy for this reason will result in a relatively minor
performance improvement. In this case there is the danger of
overloading by too intensified exercise therapy. Under these
conditions it can be observed, that the enlarged heart becomes
even larger by exercise therapy. This requires, as previously
mentioned, a marked reduction of physical activities.

Further questions were concerned with the problem, whether
the age of the patient or the length of the treatment in the
Rehabilitation Center influences the improvement of performance.

Te following Figure shows the changes of the maximal oxygen
pulse under the stated conditions. For the whole collective
of 1000 patients the performance increases by plus 11.5%. When
differentiated by age, it shows that the collective aged 50 to
69 indicates with plus 12.2% a highly significant improvement of
performance, just like the collective aged 30 to 49 with plus
10%. This then proves that a highly significant performance

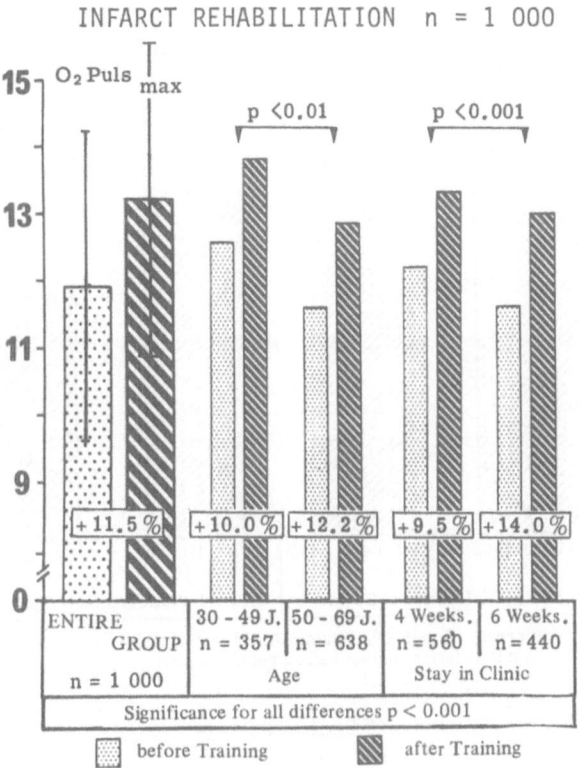

Figure 7.

improvement can be reached in a relatively short time even with
older infarct patients. On the same Figure the question is
answered, whether the performance improvement is in correlation
with the duration of the treatment. Indeed we can see, that after
6 weeks of treatment the performance improvement of plus 14% is
highly significant more pronounced than after 4 weeks of treatment
with a performance improvement of plus 9.5%.

Also of interest was the question, what about those patients
who are permitted to train at low intensity only? They show a
clear performance improvement. I have to be more detailed about
this: It is clear, that not all patients can be exercised at
the same intensity. The exercise intensity should be mainly
dependent on the size of the heart, the age of the patient, and
the results of the actually performed exercise during the in
stress test. Patients with pathologically enlarged hearts may be
exercised only at reduced intensity. Our method results initial
differentiation of exercise intensity of high, medium and low.
Patients with high intensity absolve a daily ergometer training
of 15 minutes duration with an intensity of 70% of maximal

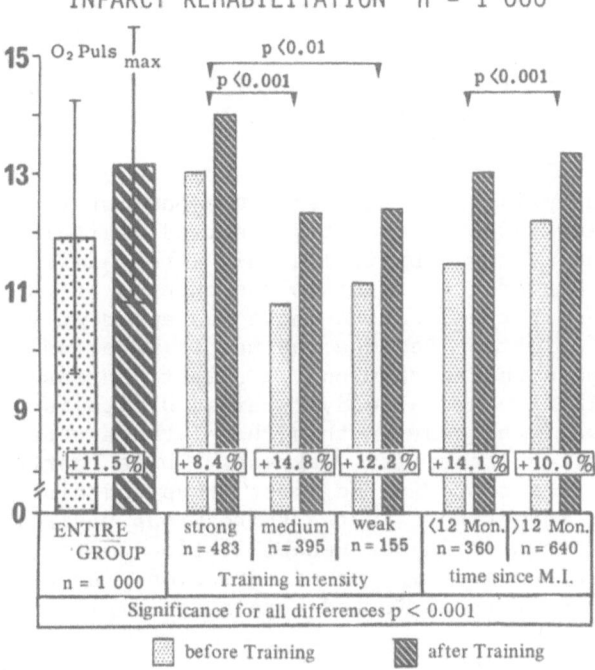

Figure 8.

performance, walks of 2 to 3 hours duration, 3 times per week.
Patients who exercise at the medium rate also exercise on the
ergometer for 15 minutes at 70%, however, they are walking only
1 to 2 hours. Low intensity patients are not permitted the
ergometer training and absolve walks of only 15 to 30 minutes.
The Figure shows again the performance improvement of the entire
collective of 1000 patients; the performance improvement is plus
11.5%. The initial performance of patients trained with high
intensity is already within a favourable range; the performance
improvement is plus 8.4% and relatively low, because the initial
working capacity was already rather high. The medium exercise
group indicates a pronounced lower initial value, as well as a
very considerable performance improvement of plus 14.8%. It is
of interest, that also the low exercise group still showed a
highly significant performance improvement of 12.2%. This result
underlines, that also low exercise intensities can still produce
highly significant performance improvement in patients after
myocardial infarction in a very short time.

Naturally the question can be asked, to what extent the
positive results in the changes of heart size and performance
are the exclusive effect of physical training, or whether, or to
what degree drugs have an influence on the hemodynamics of the

heart. Of primary consideration therefore are Digitalis and Beta-
Blockers.

    To begin with, the influence of Digitalis-therapy on the
heart size and performance is to be analysed.

    In the next Figure the total collective was divided based
on the following principle: Patients who had not received
Digitalis, patients who permanently received Digitalis, and
patients who had received Digitalis only after admission in the
Rehabilitation Center. At first to the changes of the heart
volume: In the first collective there was apparently no indication
given for Digitalization because the hearts were, on the average,
very small. These hearts show only a slight decrease in size.
The second collective had already received Digitalis during Phase
I, since apparently already in this Phase, there were grounds
for suspicion of contractility weakness. These hearts are on the
average larger than those in the first Group and also indicate a
slighly greater reduction. In the third Group Digitalization was
started after admission in our Rehabilitation Center, since the
hearts were enlarged at the time of admission. As expected, the
greatest improvement is indicated here after Digitalization.

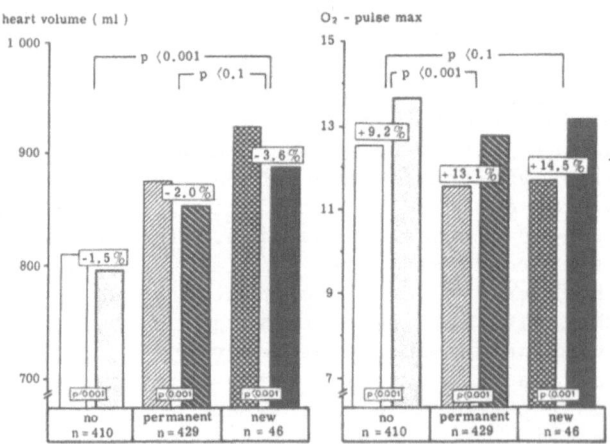

Figure 9.

Nevertheless it was established, that also for the non-digitalized Group still a significant decrease of the volume was found.

Now to the performance. As expected, in the first Group the performance was very good already before the beginning of the training, therefore no indication was given for Digitalization. Here the improvement of performance by plus 9.2% surely is sole expression of the training. In the second Group, which received Digitalis permanently, the performance increase was distinctly better, the same is true for the third Group which also was newly digitalized after admission in the Rehabilitation Center. From the result of the last 2 Groups the conclusion could be drawn, that Digitalization has produced an additional positive effect on the performance improvement besides the training effect. This is also shown by the test for significance of Group differences. Groups 2 and 3 show a significantly better performance increase than Group 1.

The following Figure analyses the question of the influence of Beta-Blockers on heart rate, maximal oxygen pulse and the heart rate - blood pressure product.

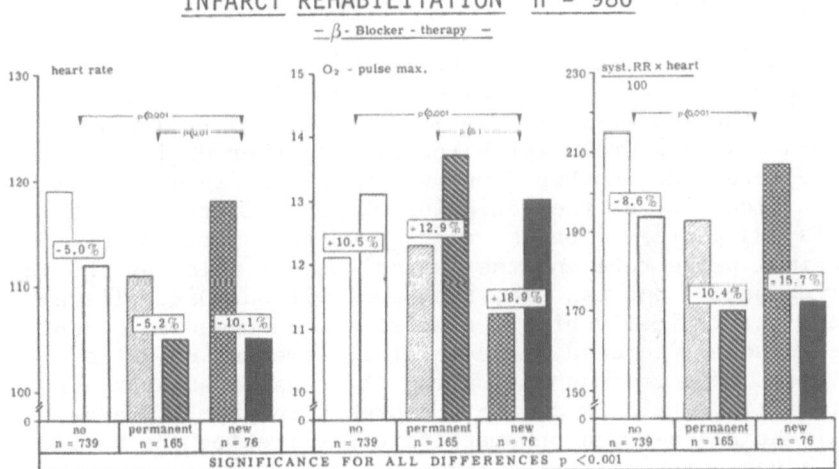

Figure 10.

At first to the pulse rate: In the first Group there are patients with relatively good initial performance. The lowering of the pulse frequency of identical sub-maximal work loads is minus 5%. The patients of the second Group were less able, were receiving B-Blockers already at the time of admission, and could be analysed only on lower sub-maximal stress levels; the mean frequencies are, for this reason, also lower than in the first Group. After training there was also a pulse reduction by 5%. The patients of the third Group showed already initially a fairly good performance capability, however, because of additional pectanginous complaints they received Beta-Blockers. This resulted in a lowering of the heart frequency by 10%. When the result of the first Group is compared with that of the third Group one can say, that the decrease of the pulse by training alone is minus 5%, that the lowering of the pulse by training plus Beta-Blockers is minus 10%, that is twice as much.

It is clear that the result of the pulse frequency indirectly also reflects in the improvement of the maximal oxygen pulse. In Group 1, without Beta-Blockers, the performance increase after training is 10.5%. In Group 3, which newly received Beta-Blockers, the performance increase is almost twice as much, plus 19%.

Similar again is the pulse - blood pressure product. The improvement of the product in the first Group, which did not receive Beta-Blockers, is minus 8.6%. The improvement in Group 3, which newly received Beta-Blockers, shows a decrease of the product by nearly 16%, again twice the amount.

This Figure indicates in summary, that through Beta-Blockers the degree of changes for the individual parameters is doubled in the same direction.

We finally examined the question, in what manner the simultaneous receipt of Digitalis and Beta-Blockers changes or influences the results. In Figure 11 the total collective was divided into a Group which received neither Digitalis nor Beta-Blockers, and another Group which had received Digitalis and Beta-Blockers, at the beginning of rehabilitation. The analysis was performed on the changes of the heart volume, the sub-maximal pulse rate and the maximal oxygen pulse as the measure of performance. One can see, that even without Digitalis and Beta-Blockers statistically highly significant changes can be obtained in the sense of decrease in heart size, lowering of pulse and improvement of performance. On the other hand, however, are the results after Digitalis and Beta-Blockers in part twice as high. The differences between pharmacologically treated and untreated Groups are statistically significant.

In closing let us pose the question, to what extent the

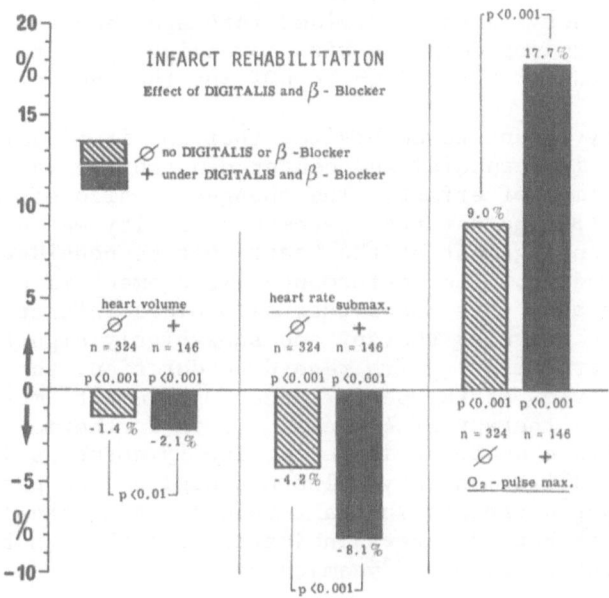

Figure 11.

performance has returned to normal after 4 to 6 weeks of treatment?
This question is best answered on the basis of the relation
between heart volume and maximal oxygen pulse. The performance
is to be considered normal, when the quotient of both values is
under 70.

INFARCT REHABILITATION   n = 1 000

TOTAL	DEPENDENT ON AGE				
	20 -29	30 - 39	40 - 49	50 - 59	60 - 69
n = 1 000					
71.3 %	100 %	85.5 %	81.3 %	66.2 %	60.6 %
n = 1 000	n = 5	n = 69	n = 288	n = 506	n = 132

Patients with normal relation between heart volume
and max.O_2 - pulse after rehabilitation.
Time since M.I. more than 3 months.

Figure 12.

The following Figure shows the percentage of those cases which had a normal relation between heart size and performance at the end of their stay at the clinic. 71% of the patients show at the end of the treatment at the Rehabilitation Clinic a normal performance. When subdivided into age decades, the rates of normal performance decrease with advancing age, starting with 100% in the youngest Group down to 60% for the ages 60 to 79.

In summary I want to emphasize, that institutional rehabilitation in a specialized center can achieve in a minimum of time an optimum of effect. The changes in size of the heart volume indicates, whether the exercise intensity was selected correctly; an enlargement of the heart must be considered as a sign of overloading. The performance improvement is not dependent upon age; this means that also older infarct patients profit from the exercise therapy and show highly significant performance improvement. With regard to duration, the 6-week therapy is, in view of the performance improvement, more effective than a therapy of 4 weeks. It is furthermore of importance, that a decrease in heart size by no means is the result of Digitalization only; also non-digitalized patients show significant decreases in heart volume. Also the analysis of the effect of Beta-Blockers indicates that these substances additionally influence hemo-dynamics decisively.

COMPARISON OF MEDICAL AND SURGICAL TREATMENT IN PATIENTS WITH

CORONARY HEART DISEASE

H. Roskamm

Benedikt Kreutz Rehabilitationszentrum
Für Herz-Und Kreislaufkranke
Bad Krozingen Ev
7812 Bad Krozingen

Coronary artery bypass grafting (CABG) is one of the most
frequent operations performed, especially in the U.S. More than 10
years after its introduction there are still discussions as to which
patients profit and which don't.

IMPROVED LIFE EXPECTANCY

Recently the discussions have centered around the results of
the Veteran-Administration Study (VA-Study). Which are the
results of this randomised study of patients with stable angina
pectoris treated from 1972 to 1974 either surgically or
conservatively - incl. beta-adrenergic blockade - over a period of
3 years?

1. Patients with a lumen narrowing of the left main stem of more
    than 50% have a significantly improved life expectancy through
    coronary heart surgery: After 3 years only 64% of the 53
    medically treated patients survived, whereas 80% of the 60
    surgically treated patients survived (32).

2. For patients with single or multiple vessel disease - excluding
    those with obstructions of the left main stem - there was no
    improvement of life expectancy through coronary heart surgery:
    after 3 years 87% of the 310 medically treated patients and 88%
    of the 286 surgically treated ones survived. This also goes
    for the various subgroups of the single-, double- and triple-
    vessel patients who have in this order a progressively worse
    prognosis (24).

This study, however, has met with massive criticism*. To mention only a few of the controversial points: relatively high operative mortality at 5.6%, relatively high frequency of perioperative infarctions at 18%, not very complete revascularis- ations (mean 1.9 grafts/patient, inspite of the fact that 86% had multiple vessel disease), relatively high bypass occlusion rate after 1 year at 31%, great frequency of those who had all grafts occluded 12%, high frequency of cross-over (17% of the patients to be treated medically were operated on during the period of observation) and brevity of the observation period: While there was no discrepancy of survival rate between medically treated or surgically treated triple-vessel patients after 3 years, a significant difference can be found in the follow-up study after 4 1/2 years: 85% of the surgically but only 76% of the medically treated group survived (27).

At the centre of discussions were questions like: why should a form of therapy be judged on the basis of mediocre results (20)? The not very favourable figures on operative mortality, frequency of perioperative infarctions and frequency of bypass occlusions might partially be a result of the fact that a great number of small hospitals with a low operations frequency and thus limited experience, was included in this study; there were 13 hospitals with a mean 22 operations in 3 years, i.e. 7 patients per year. Braunwald(4) pointed out in this respect, that these results were probably more representative of a great number of clinics where approximately 70,000 patients are operated on annually in the United States, than the excellent results of a few large centres. It should also be kept in mind that these operations were performed between 1972 and 1974 and not in 1979; the authors were able to prove that their surgical results of 1972/74 were comparable to those of the large American centres (27). The hospitals which contributed the most patients to this study - 20% - was the Veterans Administrations Hospital in Hines, Illinois where completely different results were achieved (19): Even after exclusion of left-main-stem patients significantly fewer deaths occurred in the surgically treated group of 67 patients, namely 13% as compared with 31% of the 55 conservatively treated group. In the overall comparison and evaluation of results from all participating hospitals it was surprisingly found out that the positive effect of CABG as proved in Hines was not due to a significantly worse survival rate of the medically treated patients as compared with the other hospitals.

---

*For example: Special correspondence; A debate on coronary bypass.
          New Engl. J. Med. 297:1464 (1977).

It can be expected that in the other centres patients with
enlarged hearts or bad left ventricles were excluded from the
study more readily than in Hines. At any rate, this study might
prove that results of randomization can be inconclusive. It cannot
be expected that Hines Hospital for example disregard their own good
surgical results of a randomized study in fabour of the combined
study results when to comes to the treatment of their own patients.

Randomized studies including many hospitals, always run the
risk of asserting the criteria of exclusion that cannot be measured
or numbered - such as diffuse coronary atherosclerosis, or global
ventricular insufficiency - in a non-uniform manner. In addition
to that there is the even more difficult handling of indications
for coronary angiography - in the VA-study 1461 patients out of
3659 had an angiography and of those 686 were included in the
study - the varying quality of coronary surgery plays another
important part. On the other hand it is technically and ethically
not possible for every centre to do their own randomised study,
the results of which would have validity only for that centre.

Following the VA-study several working groups in the U.S. have
compared the survival rate of their surgical patients with that of
the medically treated VA-study patients. Here it must be mentioned
that the survival rate of the medically treated VA-study patients
was significantly better than in older studies (5, 6, 17) - even
when using data according to today's criteria of operable patients
(26), whether this is due to the recent and more effective therapy,
i.e. beta-adrenergic blocking agents or due to a different
selection, remains to be seen. In these follow-up studies it was
verified that patients were comparable in all factors determining
prognosis. In this Flemma(10) was able to show that there is no
improvement of prognosis in single-vessel-disease; in double-vessel
disease there is a significant improvement (96% survivors after
4 years vs. 87%) and in triple-vessel disease a very pronounced
improvement of prognosis (93% vs. 73%).

We have similar results of Hall(14) in Houston, Texas. We
can therefore count on improved prognosis through coronary surgery
not only in left main stem disease but also in multiple-vessel-
disease, at any rate when performed in a centre with a good
surgical experience**. In this connection we find the results of

---

**Meanwhile preliminary results have been published by the European
Multicenter-Study: 2 years postop significantly more (95.9%)
patients with 3-vessel disease survived than in the conservatively
treated group (90.4%). Varnauskas E.D.: A multicenter randomised
aorto-coronary bypass study. Amer. J. Cardiol. 43:382 (Abstr.)
(1979).

Campeau(8) of importance: out of 65 patients who showed one year
after CABG optimal graft patency - each >50% stenosed vessel had
received an open bypass - 98% had survived 6 years after surgery.
Prerequisite of good long term results seems to be completeness
of revascularisation; (11a) here the VA study with 1.9 grafts per
patients and a high occlusion rate does not figure very prominently.

Another method of studying the effect of coronary surgery is
the comparison of survival curves of operated patients with
curves of normal population, age and sex relative. Considering
our knowledge of prognosis for patients with CHD it must be very
impressive to find that certain centres can produce survival
curves of their surgically treated patients up to 4 or 5 years
post-operatively, pratically identical to those of normal
population. Attention was drawn to the fact that also this method
was prone to criticism: the so called 'normal population' includes
cancer patients and people with other life-threatening disease, who
were to a great extent excluded from the surgery group (9).

Improvement of symptoms

Overall one should be very reluctant to lead the discussions
on coronary surgery merely on the basis of proven or not proven
prolongation of life expectancy. The significant effect of aorto-
coronary bypass surgery is improvement of angina pectoris in about
90% of patients. In about two-thirds of patients angina pectoris
disappears completely. Clinical improvement, when combined with
an improved exercise tolerance is, in most instances, the direct
result of revascularisation and certainly not a placebo effect.
This can be demonstrated by post-operative evaluation of exercise
tests (28), Fig. 1, myocardial lactate metabolism (31) and
scintigraphic (16) and angiographic (7) studies. Symptomatic and
functional improvement is relative to completeness of revascularisation, as can be seen angiographically (18, 30), Fig. 2. In
patients with severe angina pectoris the surgically achieved extent
of symptomatic improvement is overall much greater than by any other
conservative method (11). This improves the quality of life
considerably. The degree of symptomatic improvement declines with
time,but for the majority of patients it lasts for years (13, 30).
Symptomatic improvement is often sufficient to allow patients to
return to work. Social, economic and psychological factors often
hampter optimal rehabilitation. The longer the period of inactivity
before surgery, the less likely is a return to work. It is
certainly justified to consider in the indication for CABG the
occupational aspect, especially in patients with mild angina
pectoris.

A patient treated with the full range of conservative therapy
who cannot pursue his normal occupational activities because of

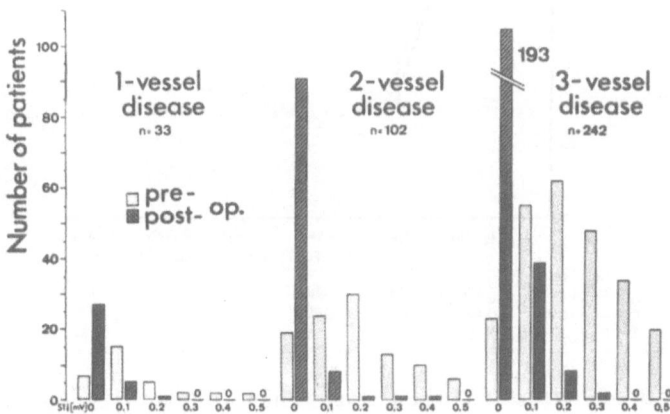

Fig. 1.   Preoperative and postoperative ST-segment depression in
relation to vessel involvement.

angina pectoris pains and at the same time offering justified
hope to be able to do so after successful CABG will certainly be
referred to surgery.

Reliable data about the effect of aortocoronary bypass surgery
on prevention of myocardial infarction are as yet not available.
The term 'prevention of myocardial infarction through CABG', so
enthusiastically accepted by the non-medical population, can as
yet not be documented, but may well be in the future, when improved
methods for myocardial protection further have reduced the incidence
of perioperative infarction.

Emergency Operation for Patients with Unstable Angina Pectoris?

The benefits of CABG on unstable angina pectoris are generally
similar to those for patients with stable angina pectoris. Data
available from a controlled study show no difference in mortality and
rate of myocardial infarction between medically and surgically
treated cases; the surgically treated ones are on a long-term

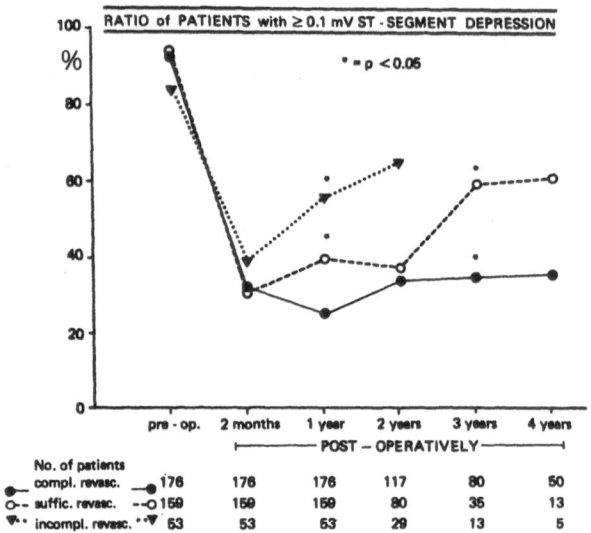

Fig. 2. Ratio of patients with more than 0.1 mV St-segment
depression in relation to completeness of revascularisation.

basis more often without their symptoms (25). Where the long term
effect is the decisive factor, surgery as well as coronary
angiography can wait. The angiogram should only be made after
medically achieved stability of angina pectoris. There is should
be pointed out that instability may well be due to a coronary spasm
occurring in a not critically stenosed vessel (21), which may in
turn be the reason for a good response to nitrates and calcium
antagonists. There is doubtless a minority of cases with instable
angina pectoris in whom intensive medical therapy may not control
symptoms of recurrent ischemia. Here a coronary angiography and
surgery may become necessary in the unstable phase. The use of an
intra-aortic balloon pump is often advisable.

Benefits of CABG in Recurrent Life-Threatening Arrhythmias?

A clear proof of the benefit of CABG in patients with recurrent
life-threatening arrhthmias (ventricular fibillation and tachycardias)
has not yet been documented. There are few reports of isolated cases
where surgery was beneficial. The effect of aneurysmectomy on
recurrent life-threatening arrhthmias will remain undiscussed here.

Indications for Coronary Artery Surgery

A working group of cardiologists and heart surgeons from Europe and the U.S.A., among them the author of this article, was convened by the WHO in Den Haag from November 1st to 4th, 1977 to distinguish between clearly established and less clearly established indications as well as contraindications (34).

A. Clearly established indications for bypass grafting are:

1. stable or unstable angina pectoris when there is an obstruction of more than 50% in the left main stem

2. stable angina pectoris, sufficient to impair substancially the individual's usual level of activity, which has not responded to adequate medical treatment over a period of at least 3 months

3. unstable angina pectoris which has not responded to conservative management

4. recurrent episodes of unstable angina pectoris

B. Less clearly established indications are:

1. mild angina pectoris in patients with multiple vessel disease

2. asymptomatic patients with stenosis of more than 50% of the left main stem

C. Contraindications are:

1. acute myocardial infarction

2. cardiac failure due to diffuse myocardial scarring without angina pectoris

3. associated terminal disease or chronic disease that will effect longevity.

Naturally there is controversy about these guidelines which represent merely the labouriously gained compromise of all members of the working group. Inter alia, the critial proximal lesion of the LAD in combination with medium angina pectoris is not mentioned among the less clearly established indications. In concurrence with a number of other centres we see especially where this vessel is concerned - several authors have reported a bad prognosis (5, 6, 17) - an indication to operate, even when there is only mild angina pectoris but when the following conditions are met: large vessel, proximal occlusion, very severe narrowing, not visible collaterals, no significant transmural myocardial infarction. For

a minority of patients in this group the mechanical method of
catheter dilatation could possibly become the best therapy. We
also think that the initial 3 months of conservative therapy in
young patients with severe stable angina pectoris, e.g. a 25
watt angina, could sometimes be a waste of time, as it is by now
well documented that angina pectoris of this degree of severity
can never be satisfactorily managed conservatively.

Surgery according to not clearly established indications should
preferably be performed only in centres with great experience (34),
where there is adequate evaluation and documentation of short-
and long-term effects of CABG. Surgical treatment of an isolated
critical lesion of the proximal part of the LAD should according
to Abedin and Dack (1) only be indicated where the surgical team
has a documented operative mortality of less than 1%, a perioperative incidence of myocardial infarction below 4% and a graft
occlusion rate of less than 10%.

The dividing line between surgical or medical therapy is
dynamic; the efficacy of new non-surgical secondary prevention has
been proved during the last few years, e.g. cessation of smoking,
beta-adrenal receptor blocking agents and probably also platelet
aggregation affecting drugs.

Medical and surgical management should complement each other in
the therapy of CHD; there is good hope for the realisation of an
effective differential therapy in the not too distant future.

SUMMARY

Medical treatment consists of elimination of risk factors,
exercise therapy, nitrates, β-blocking agents and Ca^{++} -antagonists;
surgical treatment consists of aortocoronary bypass surgery and
aneurysmectomy.

A comparison of the two can be done on three levels:

1. functional improvement; e. g. improvement of symptoms and signs
    of coronary insufficiency

2. improvement of prognosis

3. prevention of myocardial infarction

ad 1: The degree of symptomatic improvement and the increase of
exercise tolerance after successful surgery is far greater than can
be observed with any other form of treatment available to date.

ad 2: Improvement of prognosis after successful surgery can only
be achieved in specific subgroups of patients.

<u>ad 3</u>: Prevention of myocardial infarction has not been proven by either treatment.

On the basis of this comparison "clearly established" and "less clearly established" indications for aortocoronary bypass surgery will be discussed.

References

1. Z. Abedin, S. Dack, Isolated left anterior descending artery disease, Choice of therapy, Am. J. Cardiol. 40:654 (1977).
2. G. Ahlmark, und H. Saetre, Long-term treatment with beta-blockers after myocardial infarction, Eur. J. Clin. Pharmacol, 10:77 (1976).
3. Anturane Reinfarction Trial Research Group, Sulfinpyrazone in the prevention of cardiac death after myocardial infarction, N. Eng. J. Med. 298:289 (1978)
4. E. Braunwald, Coronary-artery surgery at the crossroads, N. Eng. J. Med. 297:661 (1977).
5. A. Bruschke, W. Proudfit, F. Sones, Progress study of 590 consecutive non-surgical cases of coronary disease followed 5-9 years, I. Arteriographic correlations, Circulation 47:1147 (1973).
6. G. Burgraf, J. Parker, Prognosis in coronary artery disease, Angiographic, hemodynamic and clinical factors, Circulation 51:146 (1975).
7. W.Bussmann,R. Thaler, J. Heeger, G. Kober et al: Angiographische und hämodynamische Befunde des linken Ventrikels nack Volumenbelastung und körperlicher Arbeit bei Patienten mit koronarer Herzkrankheit. Verh. Dtsch. Ges. Kreisl. Forsch. 41:168 (1975).
8. L. Campeau, Survival following aorto-coronary bypass graft surgery, in: the first decase of bypass graft surgery for coronary artery disease, (syllabus) Cleveland, September 1977, Seite 121.
9. R. Conti, Influence of Myocardial Revascularization on Survival, Am. J. Cardiol. 42:330 (1978).
10. R. J. Flemma, The effects of aortocoronary bypass surgery on life expectancy - a non-randomized study. In: H. Roskamm, M. Schmuziger (Eds.) Coronary Heart Surgery - a Rehabilitation Measure. Intl. Symposium, Bad Krozingen, 1978, im Druck, Springer, Heidelberg.
11. M. Frick, Long-term effects of coronary bypass surgery on exercise tolerance: a 2-year randomized study. In: H. Roskamm, M. Schmuziger (Eds.) Coronary Heart Surgery - a Rehabiliation Measure. Intl. Symposium, Bad Krozingen, 1978, im Druck, Springer Heidelberg.

11a. H. Gohlke, C. Gohlke, K. Schnellbacker et al, Bestimmt die
     Vollständigkeit der Revaskularisation die Erhaltung des
     funktionellen Operationseffektes bei AP-Patienten? Abstract
     45. Annual Meeting, German Soc. of Circulatory Res. April 1979

12. A. Grüntzig: Die perkutane transluminale Rekanalisation
     chronischer Arterienverschlusse mit einer neuen Dilatation-
     stechnik. Dilatation von Koronarstenosen, Verlag G. Witzstrock,
     Baden-Baden, Köln, New York, Seite 68.

13. R. Hall, G. Efrain, S. Virendra, et el: Long-term follow-up after
     coronary artery bypass. International Symposium, The First
     Decade of Bypass Graft Surgery for Coronary Artery Disease,
     September 1977, Cleveland.

14. R. Hall, Does coronary bypass surgery prolong life expectancy?
     In: H. Roskamm, M. Schmuziger (Eds.) Coronary Heart Surgery –
     a Rehabilitation Measure. Intl. Symposium, Bad Krozingen,
     1978, im Druck, Springer, Heidelberg.

15. J. Hurst, S. King, R. Logue et al: Value of coronary bypass
     surgery, Am. J. Cardiol. 42:308 (1978).

16. A. Kolibash, T. Call, R. Lewis, et.al, Myocardial perfusion
     as an indication of graft patency following coronary artery
     bypass surgery, Circulation (Abstr. 91) II 58, IV (1978).

17. P. Lichtlen, W. Steinbrunn, Complete five-year survival rates
     in 244 unselected, unoperated coronary patients undergoing
     angiography. In preparation.

18. P. Lichtlen, Liese, K. Leitz, H. Borst, Postoperative Klinik
     nack aorto-koronarem Venen-Bypass in Relation zum Ausmaß der
     Revaskularisation. Z. Kardiol. 67:83 (1978).

19. H. Loeb, A critical review of the Veterans Administration
     Cooperative study, in: Coronary Heart Surgery – a Rehabilitation
     Measure. Bad Krozingen Symposium, March 1978, im Druck bei
     Springer Heidelberg.

20. F. Loop, W. Proudfit, W. Sheldon, Coronary bypass surgery
     weighed in the Balance, Am. J. Cardiol. Eds. 42:154 (1978).

21. A. Maseri, S. Severi, M. DeNes, et al, "Variant" angina:
     one aspect of a continuous spectrum of vasospastic myocardial
     ischemia, Am. J. Cardiol. im Druck.

22. H. McIntosh, J. Garcia, the first decade of aortocoronary bypass
     grafting, 1967-1977, a review. Circulation 57, III, 405 (1978).

23. Multicentre International Study,Improvement in prognosis of
     myocardial infarction by long-term β-adrenoreceptor blockade
     using practolol. Br. med. J. III 735 (1975).

24. M. Murphy, H. Hultgren, K. Detre, J. Thomsen and T. Takara,
     Treatment of chronic stable angina, A preliminary report of
     survival data of the randomized veterans administration
     cooperative study, New Eng. J. Med. 297:621 (1977).

25. G. Plotnick, C. Conti, Unstable angina, angiography, short- and
     long-term morbidity, mortality and symptomatic status of
     medically treated patients, Am.J. Med. 63:870 (1977).

26. W. Proudfit, Minor prognostic associations, In: The first
     decade of bypass graft surgery for coronary artery disease.
     Intl. Symposium, Cleveland 1977.

27. R. Read, M. Murphy, H. Hultgran, et al, Survival of men treated for chronic stable angina pectoris, a cooperative randomized study, J. Thorac Cardiovasc Surg. 75 I, 16 (1978).

28. H. Roskamm, M. Schmuziger, K. Jauch, J. Petersen et, Ergometrische und hämodynamische Ergebnisse nack aorto-koronarer Bypass-Operation bei 378 Patienten. Schw. med. Wschr. 107 :1888 (1977).

29. H. Roskamm, P. Rentrop, A. Weisswange, Ch. Hahn, M. und Schmuziger, Improvement of ECG and haemodynamics during exercise after aorto-coronary bypass surgery. 7th European Congress of Cardiology, Amsterdam 1976.

30. P. Stürzenhofecker, H. Roskamm, K. und Schnellbacker, Factors influencing improvement of hemodynamics during exercise, Coronary Heart Surgery – a Rehabilitation Measure, H. Roskamm und M. Schmuziger, (Eds.) Intl. Symposium, Bad-Krozingen, 1978, im Druck, Springer, Heidelberg.

31. H. Swan, K. Chatterjee and E. Matloff, Alterations in ventricular mechanical and metabolic dysfunction following myocardial revascularisation in man, Ventricular Function at Rest and During Exercise, Eds. H. Roskamm and Ch.Hahn, Springer Verlag, Berlin Heidelberg New York 1976.

32. T. Takaro, H. Hultgran, M. Lipton and K. Detre The VA Cooperative Randomised Study of Surgery for Coronary Artery Occlusive Disease. II. Subgroup with Significant Left Main Lesions, Cardiovascular Surgery 1975, Supp 3, Circulation 54:107 (1976).

33. A. Vendin, C. Wilhelmsson, und L. Werkö, Chronic alprenolol treatment of patients with acute myocardial infarction after discharge from hospital, effects on mortality and morbidity, Acta med. scand. suppl. 575:1 (1975).

34. World Health Organisation, Report on a Working Group, The long-term effects of coronary bypass surgery, Den Haag, November 1977.

LONG-TERM INTERVENTION WITH BETA-BLOCKING AGENTS IN ISCHEMIC

HEART DISEASE

Lars Wilhelmsen

Department of Medicine
Östra Hospital
S-416 85 Göteborg
Sweden

Coronary heart disease (CHD) is the predominant cause of death in most industrialized countries. Sudden coronary death (SD) occuring within one hour, or, according to other definitions, within 24 hours of the onset of symptoms, has been found to be the most common type of death, both in the early phases of CHD and during several years' follow-up after a myocardial infarction (MI) (1, 2). There is reason to believe that most of these sudden deaths are due to ventricular tachyarrhythmias. In an attempt to find a basis for secondary preventive measures against CHD, it might be useful to study both risk factors both for a first and a secondary CHD event, and possible pathophysiologic mechanisms for the sudden cardiovascular catastrophe (3).

RISK FACTORS

Usually, the same risk factors are found in persons subject to nonfatal CHD as in those with fatal CHD and SD. Thus, the risk of SD has been related to smoking habits, hypertension, hypercholesterolemia, and, in some studies, to obesity, diabetes, lack of physical activity, and ECG changes (4-9); alcohol intemperance has also been associated with MI or SD (9, 10). Recent findings however, indicate more profound aberrations in those who die from CHD than in those who survive the initial attack (11).

Ventricular premature beats (VPB's) detected at rest (8) or during exercise (12) do not seem to be associated with an increased risk of MI or SD in otherwise healthy individuals; they have been found associated with increased risk in subjects with a diseased myocardium as evidenced by associated ECG abnormalities,(8, 13, 14), however, or in patients who had suffered an MI (15-18).

Mechanisms in Acute CHD

The basic problem in CHD is a reduced myocardial blood supply relative to the myocardial energy demand. Although the supply usually is reduced, the demand might be enhanced in certain circumstances, as, for example, during increased sympathetic activity. Once the myocardium becomes ischemic, its metabolism switches utilization from fat to carbohydrate, which, in turn, decreases energy production and reduces the contractile activity. The resulting reduction in mechanical performance results in dilatation of the heart and a reflex increase in sympathetic tone and, thus, a further increase in the energy demand.

A direct result of the ischemic process is a change in myocardial cell membrane integrity that rapidly leads to increased electrical excitability with a shortening of the refractory period and a lowering of the fibrillation threshold. In an infarcted myocardium, the ventricular fibrillation threshold may be reduced by about 75% (19, 20). The systemic catecholamine release induced by the acute ischemic process may further increase the suscept- ibility to arrhythmias, and certain types of arrhythmia may persist or recur long after the acute MI without intervention of a new ischemic episode (21). If the infarction can be resected, however, the fibrillation threshold may be restored to normal (22).

Pathology studies have shown that ischemic tissue damage is spotty in the periphery of the injured zone (23,24). Relatively minor alterations in the balance between energy supply and demand (e.g., increased catecholamine release, arrhythmias) at this time can influence the ultimate size of the infarcted area. Thus, factors associated with infarct size and the tendency for ventricular tachyarrhytmias to occur seem to be closely inter- related; clinical observations, for example, corroborate an association between infarct size and occurrence of VPB's in myocardial infarction (25,26).

An important question relative to attempts to prevent SD is whether it is helpful to reduce the tendency toward ventricular tachyarrhythmias, per se, or whether it is more important to ameliorate the impending imbalance between myocardial substrate demand and supply. During recent years, reports have been published indicating a favourable effect of beta-adrenergic blockade on myocardial metabolism resulting in a reduction of the extent of infarction (27-29). Beta-adrenergic blocking agents, as well as other agents that may reduce the infarct size recently reviewed by Braunwald and Maroko (24), might be most valuable in preventing serious arrhythmias in acute CHD. Beta-blocking agents have been found to greatly reduce mortality when given prior to experimental coronary occlusion, but not when given afterward(30-32).

Clinical Studies

The risk of a new CHD event is many times higher among patients who have survived an MI than in the general population, and among groups of MI patients the prognosis varies dramatically. Thus, we have found, according to multivariate prediction, that among the 10% of MI patients at greatest risk of dying within the first two years of infarction we could isolate 68% of all fatal cases (33). The increased mortality was associated with the size of the infarction, and also a history of previous MI.

Postinfarction patients, but especially those with a poor prognosis, might derive great benefit from preventive measures, and this group is very suitable for secondary preventive trials.

Amsterdam et al (34) presented preliminary results suggesting decreased mortality in a group of patients with CHD treated with propranolol. This finding, and some of the experimental findings discussed above, provided a sufficient basis for trials of beta-adrenergic blocking agents in patients who had survived MI.

After a few inconclusive studies a double-blind study was started by our group in 1970. It was found extremely useful to stratify the patients at entry to the study according to predicted risk of a new coronary event (3, 25, 35). A significant decrease in SD was found during a two-year follow-up in the group treated with alprenolol (n=114) compared with placebo (n=16), i.e. 3 deaths compared with 11 during the two years (p<.05). It was also found that two of the three patients dying suddenly in the alprenolol group had exhibited negative urinalyses for alprenolol at the two examinations immediately prior to death. The difference in the incidence of SD persisted when the total mortality in the two groups was compared, i.e. 7 cases and 14 cases, respectively, in the alprenolol and control groups.

The results of this study have now been corroborated in a second trial using alprenolol (36, 37) in which the patients were randomly allocated to a treatment group or a control group at hospital admission. The actively treated group and the control group happened to differ in size because of exclusions after entry to the trial, and the study protocol was not double-blind. The number of sudden deaths during two years' follow-up was one in the alprenolol group (n = 69) and nine in the control group (n = 93) p<.05. A significantly lower rate of nonfatal reinfarctions (4 cases and 15 cases, respectively) was found in both the alprenolol group and the control group (p<.05).

In these trials, similar preentry contraindications to beta blockade were used, namely cardiac decompensation despite treatment with digitalis and diuretics, bradycardia, atrioventricular block, chronic obstructive lung disease, systolic blood pressure below 110 mm Hg in the supine or standing position, labile diabetes treated with insulin, hepatic insufficiency or uremia, chronic alcoholism or drug addiction. The number of exclusions in the Göteborg trial were similar, in both the alprenolol and the placebo groups (35).

In a multicenter, double-blind trial using practolol started in 1972, 67 hospitals took part, with from 4 to 162 patients each; 1524 were randomly allocated to practolol and 1514 to placebo (38). Contraindications were essentially the same as those used in the two trials described above. Because of the serious adverse reactions reported with practolol (the "oculocutaneous syndrome"), this trial had to be terminated prematurely, but 330 actively treated patients and 336 placebo-treated patients were followed for two years. A significant difference was found in the incidence of SD within two hours after onset of symptoms, 30 in the practolol group compared with 52 in the palcebo group (p<.02), as well as a significant difference in the total number of cardiac deaths, 47 and 73, respectively (p<.02). A nonsignificant trend toward a reduction in nonfatal reinfarctions, 69 compared with 89 (p<.10), was also found. The difference persisted for total deaths before withdrawal of the drug (76 compared with 152), but after withdrawal the mortality became similar in the two groups (42 and 41, respectively). In this study, the beneficial effect seemed to be confined to patients with anterior infarcts and low blood pressure at entry. The study also showed a significant reduction in cardiac arrhythmias and in the incidence of angina pectoris.

Several trials with more than 10.000 patients are now under way to further study the effects of beta-blocking drugs.

Other reports have indicated an increased mortality or the occurence of infarction after withdrawal of beta-receptor blockade (39-41); these findings have been extended by a double-blind study in 20 patients performed by Miller et al(42).

Other drugs with antiarrhythmic effects, such as quinidine, procainamide, and phenytoin, as well as other, newer agents, have not been subjected to comprehensive, long-term studies of outcome after MI. Kosowsky et al (43) found only a limited reduction in VPB's with use of quinidine or procainamide and a high frequency of side effects. However, Jones et al(44) found a significant reduction in VBP's after MI during treatment with quinidine. Phenytoin was tested during one year after myocardial infarction by Lowell et al(45) who found a slight, insignificant effect on VPB frequency and no effect on mortality in 283 patients randomly allocated to active drug, compared with 285 patients given placebo.

Intervention aimed at limiting myocardial damage at the time
of the first infarct. The major secondary risk factors are all
associated with a large infarction, and it is logical to try to
limit the myocardial damage, which may be possible in the early
acute stage. Such measures might then result not only in a lower
acute mortality, but also in less invalidity as well as a better
long-term prognosis. Beta-blocking drugs will minimize the oxygen
demand, partly by decreasing the blood pressure-heart rate product,
partly by inhibiting the effect of the ischemia-induced myocardial
catecholamine release. A double-blind randomized trial of a beta-
blocker (metoprolol) given intravenously immediately after the
patient's arrival at the hospital is now going on in Göteborg with
the aim of evaluating the effects of acute beta-blockade on
infarction size, arrhythmias and the acute and long-term mortality.

DISCUSSION

Both experimental and clinical studies have indicated valuable
preventive effects against SD and MI during treatment with beta-
adrenergic blocking drugs in CHD, but purely antiarrhythmic durgs
have been of no particular value, according to data available at
present. The question arises whether all post-MI patients should
be treated with beta blockers or if this treatment should be
restricted to certain high-risk groups. In the three studies
reviewed, reductions in the total number of all cardiac events was
demonstrated. It is therefore possible that beta-blocking agents
may not only reduce the risk of sudden death but also prevent MI.
The system now available for predicting prognosis after MI is
effective only in predicting death. With the exception of continued
smoking after MI (46), the risk of a nonfatal recurrence is generally
unrelated to the same risk factors, and nonfatal reinfarction has
proved difficult to predict. The risk of both fatal and nonfatal
reinfarction is dramatically increased among patients who have
sustained a first MI. During the first year after infarction the
risk of death and reinfarction is about 30 times higher among male
infarct patients than among healthy men. Therefore, it is natural
that the pharmacologic possibilities have been tested first in post-
MI patients. It is also possible, however, that beta-blocking
drugs might be effective in improving the longevity in patients with
angina pectoris and hypertension. Such a trial in hypertension was
started by our group in 1976 involving several centers in Europe
and Canada.

Hitherto, it has been impossible to analyze in detail the
reason why beta-adrenergic blocking agents are effective. Three
mechanisms might be operative in chronic blockade; it might prevent
MI; it might prevent malignant arrhythmias in initial phase of
infarction; it might influence the size of the ischemic area.

When combined, the results of studies with beta blockers given after MI suggest that all of the three postulated modes of action are indeed plausible. Further studies are therefore needed, to elucidate the detailed mechanisms involved. Only then can the patients group be discerned in which beta-blocker treatment would be particularly beneficial. Meanwhile, it seems reasonable to recommend general beta-blocker treatment for most postinfarction patients for one to two years after infarction.

SUMMARY

Most CHD deaths are sudden, and the majority occur outside the hospital. The mechanisms are not completely known, but the basic problem in all CHD is a reduced blood supply relative to the myocardial energy demand. The ischemic process leads to a lowered fibrillation threshold and thereby increases susceptibility to arrhythmias.

Since most deaths occur soon after the onset of symptoms, therapeutic agents should, ideally, already be in use when the acute process starts. Laboratory studies have demonstrated that beta-adrenergic blocking agents administered prior to experimental coronary occlusion prevent ventricular fibrillation, in contrast with results of administration after infarction. Recent studies have suggested a similar effect in human subjects. Further controlled studies of chronic beta blockade after myocardial infarction have demonstrated a reduced sudden-death mortality during long-term follow-up. Other antiarrhythmic drugs have been of no particular value, according to the data that are available at the present time.

References

1. M. Rono, Factors related to sudden death in acute ischemic heart disease. Acta Med Scand (Suppl) 547:194 (1972).
2. B. Lown, "Sudden death from coronary heart disease. Early Phases of Coronary Heart Disease: The Possibility of Prediction". Skandia International Symposia, Stockhold, (1973) pp 255-277.
3. L. Wilhelmsen, A. Vedin, C. Wilhelmsson: Beta blockade and sudden death following myocardial infarction. Cardiovasc. Med. 3:557-563 (1978).
4. F. H. Epstein: Risk factors in coronary heart disease: environmental and hereditary influences. Isr. J. Med Sci 3:594-607 (1967).
5. Report of Inter-Society Commission for Heart Disease Resources: Primary prevention of the atherosclerotic diseases. Circulation 42:A55-95 (1970).
6. H. Blackburn, H. L. Taylor, A. Keys: Coronary heart disease in seven countries: the electrocardiogram as predictor of five-

year coronary heart disease incidence among men aged forty through fifty-nine. Circulation 41-42 (suppl 1) 154 (1970).

7. A. Vedin, C. Wilhelmsson, D. Elmfeldt, G. Tibblin, L. Wilhelmsen, L. Werkö: Sudden death: identification of high risk groups. Am Heart J. 86:124-132 (1973).

8. B. Kannel, T. Gordon:"Assessment of coronary vulnerability. Early Phases of Coronary Heart Diseases: The Possiblity of Prediction". Skandia International Symposia, Stockholm (1973) p.123.

9. L. Wilhelmsen, H. Wedel, G. Tibblin: Multivariate analysis of risk factors for coronary heart disease. Circulation 48:950-958 (1973).

10. D. Elmfeldt, A. Vedin, C. Wilhelmsson, Tibblin, L. Wilhelmsen, Morbidity in representative male survivors of myocardial infarction compared to representative pupulation samples. J. Chronic Dis. 29:221-231 (1976).

11. G. Tibblin, L. Wilhelmsen, L. Werkö: Risk factors for myocardial infarction and death due to ischemic heart disease and other causes. Am J Cardiol. 35:514-522 (1975).

12. B. W. Chiang, L. V. Perman, L. Ostrander, F. Epstein: Relationship of premature systoles to coronary heart disease and sudden death in the Tecumseh epidemiologic study. Ann Intern Med. 70:1159-1166 (1969).

13. A. Vedin, C. Wilhelmsson, L. Wilhelmsen, B. Ekström-Jodal, J. Bjure: The relationships of resting and exercise induced ectopic beats to other ischemic manifestations and to coronary risk factors. Am J Cardiol. 30:25-31 (1972).

14. L. Wilhelmsen, G. Tibblin, M. Aurell, J. Bjure, B. Ekström-Jodal, G. Grimby,: Physical activity, physical fitness and risk of myocardial infarction. Adv. Cardiol. 18:217-230 (1976).

15. A. J. Moss, J. De Camilla, F. Engström, W. Hoffman, C. Odoroff, H. Davis,: The posthospital phase of myocardial infarction: identification of patients with increased mortality risk. Circulation 49:460-466 (1974).

16. Coronary Drug Project Research Group: Prognostic importance of premature beats following myocardial infarction: Experience in the coronary drug project. JAMA 223:1116-1124 (1973).

17. M. N. Kotler, B. Tabatznik, M. M. Mower, S. Tominage: Prognostic significance of ventricular ectopic beats with respect to sudden death in the late postinfarction period. Circulation 47:959-966 (1973).

18. L. A. Vismara, E. A. Amsterdam, D. T. Mason,: Relation of ventricular arrhythmias in the late hospital phase of acute myocardial infarction to sudden death after hospital discharge. Am. J. Med. 59:6-12 (1975)

19. N. E. Shunway, J. A. Johnson, R. J. Stish: The study of ventricular fibrillation by threshold determinations. J. Thorac Surg. 34:643 (1957).

20. C. M. Phibbs, R. A. van Tyn, L. D. McLean: Vulnerability of the dog heart to ventricular fibrillation: A comparative study

of chronic ischemia and three myocardial revascularization
procedures. J. Thorac Cardiovasc. Surg. 42:228-235 (1961).

21. B. Lown, M. Wolf: Approaches to sudden death from coronary
heart disease. Circulation 44:130 (1971).

22. S. Sakaibara, H. Hiratsuka, Y. Ota, H. Gomi, M. Yokoyama,
T. Akimoto, K. Kishi: An elevation of ventricular fibrillation
threshold after surgical resection of infarcted myocardium.
Am. Heart J. 74:381-386 (1967).

23. D. L. Page, J. B. Caulfield, J. A. Kastor, R. W. DeSanctis,:
Myocardial changes associated with cardiogenic shock. N.
Engl. J. Med. 285:133-137 (1971).

24. E. Braunwald, P. R. Maroko: The reduction of infarct size –
an idea whose time (for testing) has come. Circulation
50:206-209 (1974).

25. C. Wilhelmsson, A. Vedin, L. Wilhelmsen, G. Tibblin: Reduction
of sudden deaths after myocardial infarction by treatment with
alprenolol. Lancet 2:1157-1159 (1974).

26. R. Roberts, A. Husain, H. D. Ambos, G. C. Oliver, J. R. Cox Jr.
B. E. Sobel: Relation between infarct size and ventricular
arrhythmia. Br.Heart J. 37:1169-1175 (1975).

27. P. R. Maroko, P. Libby, J. W. Covell, B. E. Sobel, J. Ross Jr.,
E. Braunwald: Precordial ST segment elevation mapping: an
atraumatic method for assessing alterations in the extent of
myocardial interventions. Am J. Cardiol. 29:223-230 (1972).

28. J. Pelides, D. W. Reid, M. Thomas, J. P. Shillingford:
Inhibition by beta-blockade of the ST segment elevation after
acute myocardial infarction in man. Cardiovasc Res. 6:295-
301 (1972).

29. R. C. Leinback. H. K. Cold, M. J. Buckley, G. W. Austen,
C. A. Saunders: Reduction of myocardial injury during acute
myocardial infarction by early application of intra-aortic
balloon pumping and propranolol (abstract). Circulation
48 (suppl.4): 100 (1973).

30. B. I. Pentecost, G. W. Austen: Beta-adrenergic blockade
in experimental myocardial infarction. Am. Heart J. 72:790
(1966).

31. M. I. Khan, J. T. Hamilton, G. W. Manning,: Protective effect
of beta adrenoceptor blockade in experimental coronary
occlusion in conscious dogs. Am J. Cardiol. 30:832-837 (1972).

32. G. J. Kelliher, C. Widmer, J. Roberts: Seventh annual meeting
of the international study group for research in cardiac
metabolism. Abstract No.141, Quebec (1974).

33. A. Vedin, L. Wilhelmsen.H. Wedel, B. Pettersson, C. Wilhelmsson,
D. Elmfeldt, G. Tibblin: Prediction of cardiovascular deaths
and nonfatal reinfarctions after myocardial infarction.
Acta Med Scand. 201:309-316 (1977).

34. E. A. Amsterdam, S. Wolfson, R. Gorlin: Effect of therapy on
survival in angina pectoris. Ann Intern Med. 68:1151 (1968).

35. J. A. Vedin, C. Wilhelmsson, G. Tibblin, L. Wilhelmsen.

L. Werkö: Chronic alprenolol treatment of patients with acute myocardial infarction after discharge from hospital. Acta Med Scand (Suppl) 575:9–24 (1975).

36. G. Ahlmark, H. Saetre, M. Korsgren: Reduction of sudden deaths after myocardial infarction. Lancet 2:1563 (1974).

37. G. Ahlmark. H. Saetre, : Long-term treatment with beta-blockers after myocardial infarction. Eur J Clin Pharmacol. 10:77–83 (1976).

38. K. G. Green,: Improvement in prognosis of myocardial infarction by long-term beta-adrenoreceptor blockade using practolol. Br Med J., 3:735–740 (1975).

39. R. G. Diaz, J. Somberg, E. Freeman, B. Levitt: Withdrawal of propranolol and myocardial infarction. Lancet 1:1068, (1973).

40. R. Slome: Withdrawal of propranolol and myocardial infarction. Lancet 1:156 (1973).

41. E. L. Alderman, J. Coltart, G. E. Wettack, et al: Coronary artery syndromes after sudden propranolol withdrawal. Ann Intern Med., 81:625–627 (1974).

42. R. R. Miller , H. G. Olsson, E. A. Amsterdam, et al: Propranolol withdrawal rebound phenomenon. N. Eng. J. Med., 293:416–418 (1975).

43. B.D. Kosowsky, J. Taylor, B. Lown, R. F. Ritchie,: Long-term use of procaine amide following acute myocardial infarction Circulation 47:1204–1210 (1973)

44. D. T. Jones, W. J. Kostuk, R. W. Gunton: Prophylactic quinidine for the prevention of arrhythmias after acute myocardial infarction. Am J Card., 33:655–660 (1974).

45. R. R. H. Lowell, et al: Phenytoin after recovery from myocardial infarction. Lancet 2:1055–1057 (1971).

46. C. Wilhelmsson, J. A. Vedin, D. Elmfeldt, G. Tibblin, L. Wilehlmsen: Smoking and myocardial infarction. Lancet 1:415–420 (1975).

PATIENT AND FAMILY EDUCATION: A REQUISITE COMPONENT OF

COMPREHENSIVE REHABILITATION AFTER MYOCARDIAL INFARCTION

Nanette Kass Wenger

Emory University School of Medicine
Atlanta
Georgia

Illness is best controlled when the patient participates in disease management. The goal of patient and family education is to provide adequate information about the cardiac illness and its management to enable the patient to assume some responsibility for his or her continuing health care. Educational efforts are designed to identify areas of patient decision and responsibility. Dr. Lawrence Weed has said, "the most powerful of all medical and paramedical personnel is the patient - highly motivated, not costing anything - even willing to pay - and there is one for every member of the population." The effects of incorporating the patient into the health care team include a decrease in the feeling of helplessness in dealing with the cardiac problem, aid in restoring self-esteem after an illness such as myocardial infarction which constitutes a life crisis, an increased confidence of the patient in a successful outcome and an increase in the patient's ability to cope with illness. The educational programme should be instituted during the hospitalization for myocardial infarction and/or coronary bypass surgery and continued in the physician's office or in a hospital or community clinic.

An episode of myocardial infarction or coronary bypass surgery constitutes a crisis in the lives of the patient and family; motivation for learning is optimal at this time, and the hospital setting provides the opportunity for education by health care professionals. Effective teaching also requires documentation of the educational component of patient care in the patient record. At Grady Memorial Hospital and the Emory University School of Medicine in Atlanta, Georgia, an educational algorithm (Table 1) for myocardial infarction is incorporated in the patient record. It delineates the information to be presented at each stage of the

TABLE I   PATIENT EDUCATION PROGRAMME COMPONENTS*
               Problem: Myocardial Infarction

I.   Adjustment to coronary care unit
     A.   Purpose of coronary care unit
     B.   Regulations of unit (visiting, smoking, flowers)
     C.   Monitor (sounds and leads)
     D.   Intravenous infusions and medications
     E.   Oxygen
     F.   Activity (leg exercise, etc.)
     G.   ECG, blood tests, x-rays
     H.   Diet
     I.   Personal emergencies (e.g. financial, job)
II. Adjustments to transfer from unit
     A.   Constant observation no longer necessary
     B.   Activity as prescribed
     C.   Plan for education programme (see III)
III. Information needed for adaptation to disease
     A.   Normal anatomy and function of heart
     B.   Development of coronary atherosclerotic heart disease
     C.   Heart attack
          I.   Risk factors
               (a) General discussion
               (b) Emphasis on risk factors of individual patient
          2.   Warning signs of heart attack
          3.   Healing relation to physical activity
     D.   Personal response to myocardial infarction
          1.   Group discussion
          2.   Individual conference with patient, family
IV. Plans for care after discharge from hospital
     A.   Diet
          1.   Group discussion
          2.   Individual conference with patient, family
     B.   Discharge medications (each medication, its dosage, is
          listed for teaching to patient)
     C.   Activity
          1.   General
          2.   Sexual
          3.   Work simplification
     D.   Symptoms which should be reported
     E.   Rehabilitation exercises
     F.   Clinic or physician appointments
     G.   Community resources
V.   Other areas for teaching (e.g. pacemaker, diabetes
VI. Educational materials given to patient (a basic pamphlet list
     is checked and additional educational materials are recorded)
VII. Outpatient (clinic) education
     A.   Review of IV. in class and individual instruction
     B.   Patient self-learning tapes and slide tapes

*For each item listed, the date of teaching and instructor's name
are recorded as is the need for further patient education on that
topic and the instructor's comments regarding the patient's
comprehension.

Reproduced from Wenger, N.K. and Gilbert, C.A. "Rehabilitation
of the Myocardial Infarction Patient." The Heart, edited by
J. W. Hurst, McGraw-Hill, New York, 4th ed., 1978, p.1308.

illness and allows identification of the individual performing
the teaching and that person's assessment of patient learning and
learning needs. This format assures that all requisite information
is transmitted to the patient without inadvertant omissions, it
avoids unnecessary duplication of teaching efforts, but enables
repetition and reinforcement when required. The in-hospital
teaching programme forms the cornerstone for subsequent ambulatory
care educational efforts. Because patient and family education for
a chronic disease must be a long-term process, this continuity of
the educational programme is important.

     Very simple brief facts are presented in the Coronary Care
Unit, when fear, pain, anxiety and fatigue impair the physical and
mental readiness for learning. Even if this information is not
retained or remembered on a long-term basis, it provides reassurance
to both patient and family. The diagnosis is briefly explained, as
well as the reasons for and the safety features of the Coronary
Care Unit procedures and equipment; this information decreases the
likelihood that the patient will misinterpret staff actions or
comments, and helps the patient adjust to a life-threatening
situation. The temporary nature of all restrictions is emphasied,
delineating that decreased surveillance and intensity of care will
become appropriate as recovery progresses. A realistically
positive attitude of all staff members is of major value,
transmitting to the patient and family their confidence that the
patient will survive and recover to resume a normal or near-
normal lifestyle.

     More detailed educational efforts are appropriate during the
remainder of the hospitalization, when the patient is generally
pain free, has less anxiety about immediate survival, and becomes
concerned with planning for return home. The patient's needs are
a major determinant of the effectiveness of an educational
programme; information must be designed to solve what the patient
perceives as relevant problems. While individual teaching is
requisite for specific patient concerns and problems, we have found
major benefit to the class or group educational format. This
approach is economical of professional time, enables patients to
interact with and share experiences with a peer group confronting

similar problems, and reinforces the learning process by group
discussion and questions. Patients appear less anxious and self-
conscious in a group educational setting with the peer group
serving to facilitate adaptation to stress, decrease frustration
and thus enhance and reinforce learning. Effective learning
requires participation; the opportunity to function as a group
member in realistic problem-solving and to help others is also
supportive of the patient's self-esteem.

It is also necessary to define the professionals' roles in
patient and family education. The physician's major responsibility
is delineation of the educational curriculum, as well as periodic
review of instructional content to assure accuracy and timeliness.
Other health professionals - nurses, dietitians, occupational and
physical therapists, social workers, etc. - may share in the
development of teaching materials and the actual implementation of
the educational programme; typically they have the opportunity for
more prolonged contact with the patient and family.

Patients must understand their disease. For the coronary
patient this includes a brief review of normal cardiac structure
and function of the atherosclerotic process leading to coronary
obstruction, and of the changes which occur with myocardial
infarction, emphasizing the healing process. Without this background, the patient is unlikely to appreciate how coronary arterial
obstruction can cause the pain that has been experienced and how
associated disturbances of cardiac rhythm and/or of myocardial
pumping function can produce other symptoms. This teaching also
provides the basis for recommendations for care: risk factor
modification, diet, activity, medical and/or surgical therapy, etc.
Since most interventions in the management of the post-infarction
patient entail a modification of lifestyle, the teaching emphasis
should provide insight into those habits which may alter the risk
of infarction and into the value of lifestyle changes. The
rationale for dietary alterations - calories, fat, sodium - should
be presented and implementation materials and methods offered.
Specific inquiries about food preferences and eating habits enable
the delineation of a reasonable diet with enough familiar foods to
make adherence likely. Presentation of guidelines for restaurant
eating and recommended changes in food purchasing and preparation
further encourage compliance; the essential individual to be
educated is the one responsible for food preparation. The factual
basis for recommendations for cessation of cigarette smoking should
be discussed and patients referred to anti-smoking programmes in
the hospital or community. The reasons for the initial activity
restriction should be explained, with recommendations for
increasing physical activity related to myocardial healing; again,
delineation of exercise programmes and facilities within the
community is appropriate to enable the patient to implement the

physical activity recommendations. Resumption of sexual activity should also be discussed, using as a general guideline that this is appropriate when other usual daily living activities are re-instituted. Patients and their families should also be made aware of other community resources which are available when needed – counselling services, home-care agencies, vocational rehabilitation and guidance services, community post-coronary educational groups or clubs, etc. Patients and their families should also be cautioned about problems commonly encountered when the patient returns home – problems of overprotection by the family, problems related to employer and community attitudes toward myocardial infaction patients.

Patients must be taught about each medication to be taken after discharge from the hospital – its name, purpose, dosage, desired effects and untoward effects to be reported to the physician. The appropriate response to new or recurrent symptoms should be reviewed, particularly the response to chest pain, with emphasis on seeking immediate medical care for increased or prolonged chest discomfort; this approach may help decrease the pre-hospital deaths from recurrent infarction. Recently, many hospital centres have begun cardiopulmonary resuscitation instruction for family members of myocardial infarction survivors, a programme which has elicited an amazingly positive response.

Audiovisual materials enhance learning and provide a more varied and interesting educational presentation; take-home materials (books, pamphlets, instruction sheets) should be prepared for the patient to reinforce the information presented during the hospitalization. Written specific instructions provide valuable reference material and help minimize patient-family homecoming conflicts that may derive from vague or ambiguous directions or recommendations. Patient self-tests, as part of audiovisual or printed presentations, often reinforce learning when a trained professional is available to respond to the patient's questions or concerns.

In all teaching encounters a positive attitude of the health professionals is essential in helping the patient maintain self-esteem while making reasonably realistic plans for resuming or altering the prior lifestyle following a cardiac illness or cardiovascular surgery. The staff should convey their concern for the patient as an individual, their respect for the patient, and the fact that in teaching they are conferring responsibility for care on the patient.

Despite this intensive initial educational approach, repetition is needed after the patient returns home. Even if the patient has assimilated the cognitive material, the recommended changes in habit and life style must be reviewed by the patient, evaluated, and

finally incorporated into the patient's own value system; only
then can behavioral change be effected. Although the objective
of patient-family education is to effect a change in the health
related behaviour of the learner, there are three major stages in
this learning process: the first is the cognitive stage, the
information the patient must have and understand (but the information
must be perceived as meaningful and relevant to be assimilated);
the next is the affective stage, the personal value to the patient
of recommended changes and the decision as to whether or not they
can be incorporated into the newly reorganized lifestyle; and
finally, the behavioural stage involving actual implementation by
the patient. Health care professionals can provide the background
information, increase motivation by education, help the patient
acquire the skills necessary for change, help the patient set
realistic goals and offer continuing encouragement and support for
successful change, and encourage the maintenance of health-related
behaviour, but it is the patient who must function as the agent for
change.

        Is patient education of value? There is increasing evidence
that patients who understand their disease and the rationale for
the components of its management have both an increased motivation
and improved ability to adhere to health care regimens. Since
management of the post-myocardial infarction and/or post-coronary
bypass surgical patient involves lifetime care patterns, intensive
serial educational efforts appear appropriate.

References

1. N. T. Argondizzo: Patient and Family Education. In N. K.
    Wenger, H. R. Hellerstein (eds.): Rehabilitation of the
    Coronary Patient, John Wiley & Sons, Inc., New York, 1978,
    p.117.
2. C. A. Baden: Teaching the coronary patient and his family.
    Nurs Clin North Am., 7:563, (1972).
3. J. Camp, S. Vycital: Your Pacemaker. Cardiac Clinic –
    Grady Memorial Hospital, Atlanta, Georgia, (1975).
4. J. M. Dunbar: Adherence to medication: An intervention study
    with poor adherers. Circulation, 56 (Suppl 3):169, (1977).
5. V. Haferkorn: Assessing individual learning needs as a
    basis for patient teaching. Nurs Clin North Am., 6:199,
    (1969).
6. B. J. Linde, N. M. Janz: The effectiveness of a comprehensive
    teaching program on the knowledge and compliance of cardio-
    vascular patients. Circulation 56 (Suppl 3):146, (1977).
7. H. MacDaniel: Foods – To Eat to Reduce the Risk of Heart
    Attack. Cardiac Clinic – Grady Memorial Hospital, Atlanta,
    Georgia, (1974).

8. F. Mount, M. W. MacDonald: Now That Your Heart is Healing ...
    Let's Get Ready to Go Home. Cardiac Clinic - Grady
    Memorial Hospital, Atlanta, Georgia, (1973).

9. B. K. Redman: The Process of Patient Teaching in Nursing
    (ed 3). C. V. Mosby, St. Louis, (1977).

10. J. S. Smith: High Blood Pressure "The Silent Killer."
    Cardiac Clinic - Grady Memorial Hospital, Atlanta, Georgia,
    (1975).

11. K. Smyth: Teaching patients. Nurs Clin North Am., 6:571,
    (1971).

12. N. K. Wenger: Post myocardial infarction patient and family
    education. Postgrad Med., 57:129, #7, (1975).

13. N. K. Wenger, Z. F. Mount: An educational algorithm for
    myocardial infarction. Cardiovasc Nursing, 11:10, (1975).

SELECTED TOPICS IN EXERCISE ELECTROCARDIOGRAPHY

R. Messin

Laboratory of Cardio-Pulmonary Physiology and
Department of Cardiology
Hôspital Universitaire Saint-Pierre
Bruxelles, Belgium

Exercise testing with continuous monitoring and recording
of the electrocardiogram has proven to be a very useful tool
for the diagnosis of coronary insufficiency in the presence of
a typical chest pain or in coronary patients with normal resting
ECG, which happens in about one-third of the cases. A
satisfactory sensitivity of about 60% (i.e. about 40% of false
negative results) is obtainable (1), especially if loading is
sufficiently heavy, if ECG is recorded during the test as well as
during the recovery period and if analysis takes into account not
only the quantitative amount of ST changes but also the speed at
which the ST segment comes back from the J point to the baseline
(5). Moreover, specificity is at least 90% (i.e. about 10% of
false positive results) (1) if some well known factors influencing
ECG response to exercise, e.g. digitalis or electrolyte
disturbances, are recognized.

Nevertheless, some exercise ECG patterns may raise difficulties
for interpretation, a few of which will be reviewed here.

1.   Wolff-Parkinson-White(WPW) Syndrome

When Wolff and White in Boston and Parkinson in Great Britain
described the pre-excitation syndrome in 1930, they stressed
the fact that, at first examination, one-third of the cases
were misdiagnosed bundle branch block, ventricular hypertrophy,
ventricular tachycardia or myocardial infarction. They
recognized also the high incidence of false positive exercise
tests, resulting in a wrong diagnosis of coronary insufficiency.
Since that time, several authors have described ECG changes in

the WPW syndrome similar to that observed when coronary insufficiency
is present.

Very often, however, it is hard to be sure that the result
of an exercise test is a false postive one, except if intermittent
WPW syndrome is present during or after the test. As an example
(4), the history of a 45 year old man is reported. The patient
had stopped working owing to chest pain. Resting ECG showed an
intermittent WPW syndrome. During and immediately after the
exercise test, ST-T changes simulating coronary insufficiency
occured only for those complexes which showed the pre-excitation
phenomenon and no pain occured. The patient went back to work
and was retested one year later. The WPW syndrome was now
permanent at rest but became intermittent during exercise showing,
as before, ST-T changes only in complexes with the pre-excitation
syndrome. During the recovery period, however, the WPW phenomenon
reappeared constantly, with the same ST-T alterations as those
observed one year earlier(Figures 1 & 2).

SUMMARY

   a) patients with the WPW syndrome show often ECG changes
       during exercise similar to that observed when coronary
       insufficiency is present;

   b) only ECG complexes without the pre-excitation syndrome
       are liable to a correct interpretation,

   c) the disappearance of the pre-excitation syndrome during
       exercise and during the recovery period being unpredictable,
       the ECG must be necessarily recorded continuously, during
       and after effort. In the case we presented, exercise
       promoted the disappearance of the delta wave while the
       increased vagal tone of the post-exercise period made it
       to reappear.

2.   Exercise Testing in Women

   Interpretation of exercise tests is usually much more
difficult in women than in men. First, it is well known that if
heart rate does not raise enough during the test, the latter may
not be correctly interpreted, because a too small fraction of the
so-called coronary reserve has been explored. Now, in women exercise
test are often stopped prematurely, owing to a lack of motivation
to perform an effort of unusual intensity and to a lack of
muscular training; obesity can play an additional unfavourable
role. In our experience (2), this is the case for 16% of the
tests performed in women, making the decision between true and
false negative responses practically impossible; in men, on
the contrary, 5% only of the tests are uninterpretable for the

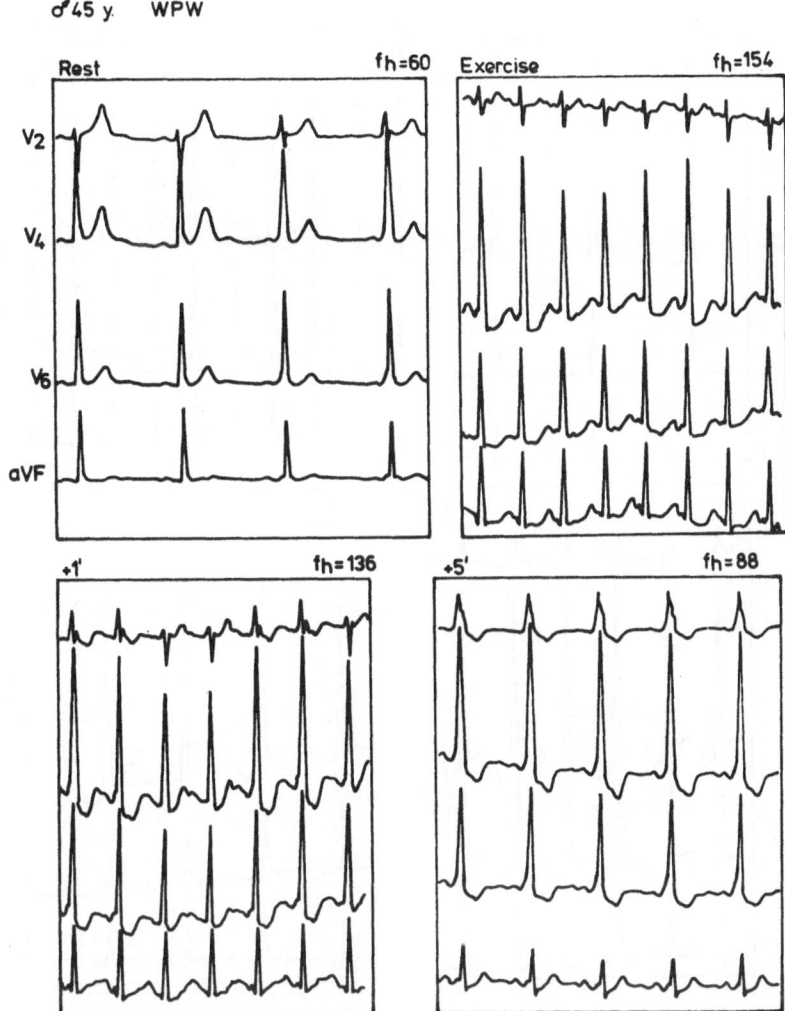

Fig. 1. Wolff-Parkinson-White syndrome in a 45 year old man. The
         pre-excitation phenomenon is intermittent at rest, during
         exercise and immediately thereafter but is constant at
         the 5th minute of the recovery period. Exercise-
         induced ST-T changes simulating coronary insufficiency
         occur only in the complexes showing abnormal conduction.
         f_h = heart rate.

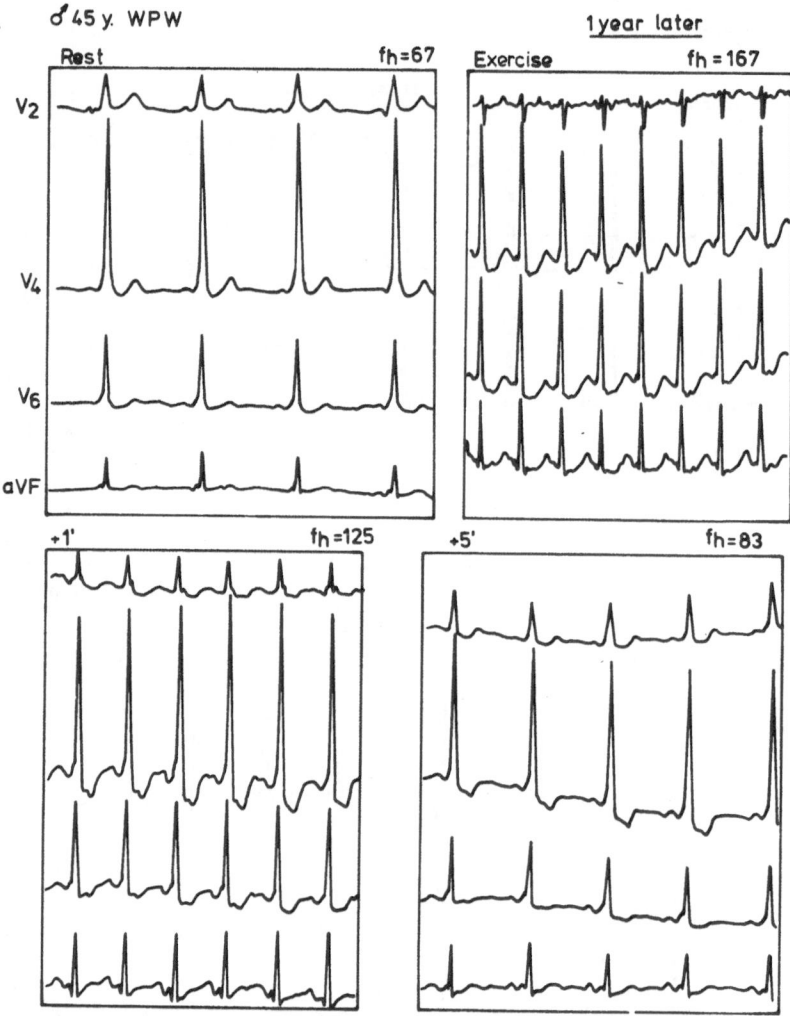

Fig. 2.   Same patient as in Figure 1, one year later.   The
          Wolff-Parkinson-White syndrome is now constant at rest
          and after exercise but is intermittent during effort.
          Exercise-induced ST-T changes observed in the complexes
          with abnormal conduction have the same features as in
          Figure 1.

          f_h = heart rate.

same reasons. Secondly, even when testing is correctly
conducted, more electrocardiographic abnormalities are observed
at rest and during exercise in women than in men, even though the
incidence of coronary disease is almost four times less in
women: .9% against 3.4% (6). Those abnormalities involve not
only T wave changes but also ST alterations suggesting sometimes
ischaemic patterns. They are more frequent with increasing age
but have usually a good prognosis.

Comparisons between coronary angiograms and exercise tests
have shown that the percentages of false positive results are
lower when resting ECG is normal (5.5 to 14%) than when it is
altered (22 to 67%). The differences between authors can be
partly explained by differences in angiographic and electrocardiographic criteria. Anyway, those percentages are higher than
for men (2 to 10%).

We performed a study in 253 males and 31 females with symptoms
who underwent an exercise test on the bicycle ergometer, the
target heart rate representing 80% of the maximal heart rate
corrected for age, as well as a selective coronary angiography, a
stenosis of at least 70% on one or more vessels being considered
as significant.

Doubtful exercise ECG changes (i.e. horizontal ST depression
less than .1 mV or unsloping ST segment showing a depression less
than .1 mV, .08 sec after its origin J) being taken into account,
we observed a sensitivity not very different in men and women,
(respectively 73% and 88%) but a much lower specificity in the
latter (respectively 88% and 55%).

Several hypotheses try to explain the high percentage of
false positive responses observed in women on exercise:

- role of oestrogens, owing to the similarity of their
  chemical structure to that of digitalis;

- abnormalities of oxyhaemoglobin dissociation curve;

- distal coronary vessels lesions;

- use of hormonal contraceptives, which are known to favour
  thromboembolism;

- manifestations of vaso-regulatory asthenia, which is more
  frequent in women, in such cases, propranolol administrated
  prior to the test would normalize many tracings (2).

SUMMARY

   a) ECG changes on exercise associated with chest pain are
       rather frequent in women with increasing age and one
       should be very cautious in making a diagnosis of coronary
       insufficiency when other proofs are lacking;

   b) most of such cases have a good prognosis: besides the
       fact that the overall incidence of myocardial infarction
       is four times less in females than in males, follow-up
       studies of women with ECG abnormalities on exercise
       have shown that myocardial infarction and sudden death
       are quite uncommon in that population.

3.   ST Segment Elevation on Exercise

The occurrence of ST segment elevation during exercise in
coronary patients with no electrocardiographic signs of previous
myocardial infarction corresponds to a severe transmural ischaemia
we call "inverted coronary insufficiency" (7). However, this
may be due to several pathological conditions, differing from
each other by their evolutive aspects as well as by the corresponding
coronary alterations which range from severe 1- or 2- to 3-vessel
lesions to a localized and reversible spastic phenomenon.

Clinical patterns: ST segment elevation on exercise may be
recorded in patients with stable effort angina lasting for many
months or years. It is more frequently seen in those with recent
chest pain getting steadily worse or occurring at rest, especially
during night.

Angiographic patterns: inverted coronary insufficiency on
exercise may be observed in cases showing severe narrowing
($\geqslant$70%) or obstruction, proximally or distally located in one
(usually the anterior descending coronary artery) or several
vessels, as well as in cases with nonsignificant coronary
lesions not justifying any surgical by-pass.

Electrocardiographic patterns: inverted coronary insufficiency
on effort is characterized by elevation of the ST segment in some
leads, associated with ST depression in opposite leads, by
heightening of the R wave, widening of the QRS complex and
occurrence of malignant arrhythmias. Sometimes, ST elevation
appears after some ST depression. Such an evolution (which can
also be observed at rest) suggests that, in those cases,
subendocardial ischaemia preceded more severe transmural
ischaemia. For that reason, whenever ST depression disappears
suddenly during exercise testing the latter should be stopped
immediately, owing to the risk that malignant arrhythmias would

develop in presence of inverted coronary insufficiency. Those
arrhythmias consist in ventricular premature beats appearing
sometimes early with changing morphology, or in multifocal
ventricular tachycardia.

Prinzmetal's syndrome, previously described as a spontaneous
access of angina with ST segment elevation, occuring in coronary
patients with a severe one-vessel lesion and possibly due to a
spastic mechanism, is merely a particular case of inverted
coronary insufficiency. The spontaneous character of the access
implies that it occurs without any change in the factors
determining myocardial oxygen requirements(i.e. telediastolic
heart volume, arterial blood pressure, heart rate, cardiac output
and contractility). In fact, angina at rest or during night is
often provoked by a light effort, emotion or dreaming so that
spontaneity of the attack can be ascertained only if this is not
preceeded by any change in heart rate during dynamic electrocardiographic recording. The role of angiospasm will be suggested
by the really spontaneous character of the anginous attack, or
by the fact that ECG response to repeated exercise tests is not
reproducible (which is different from usual coronary insufficiency),
myocardial ischaemia being in particular more severe for a
lower work load (Figure 3). Moreover, angiospasm can be induced
during coronary angiography, by intravenous injection of ergonovin (7)

SUMMARY

   a) ST segment elevation on exercise is a sign, when no
       previous myocardial infarction is present, of severe
       transmural myocardial ischaemia due to angiospasm with
       or without coronary disease (more particularly in
       connection with the Prinzmetal's syndrome), or due to
       major alterations of one of several coronary vessels,
       sometimes with poor collateral circulation;

   b) malignant arrhythmias being quite frequent when inverted
       coronary insufficiency is present, one should be aware
       of the following points:

       - exercise testing will be performed most cautiously
          if chest pain appeared recently, if angina seems to
          occur spontaneously or if it is unconstantly related
          to effort.

       - the sudden disappearance of ST depression during
          exercise requires that the test should be stopped
          immediately, because of the risk that ST elevation
          would develop quickly thereafter.

♂ 41 y ;(+ β-blockers)
angina ; f$_h$ = 110

100 W (3 mn)   +2 mn

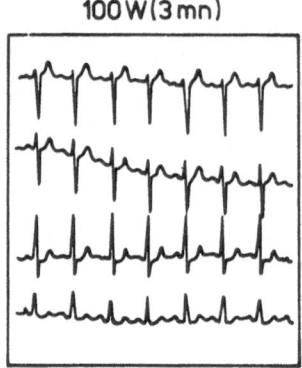 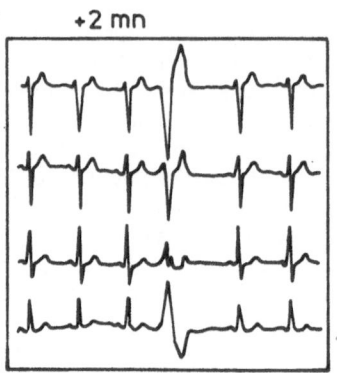

One week later (no β-blockers)
angina ; f$_h$ = 114 (75 W 2′ 15″)

+2 mn

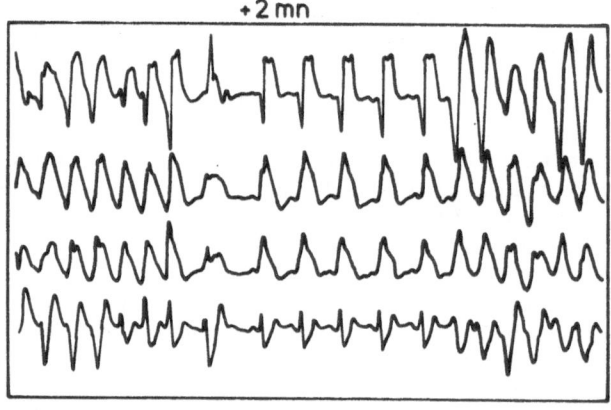

Fig. 3.   41 year old man. A load of 100 watts (performed under
β-blockers) is stopped after 3 minutes, owing to angina
plus ST segment depression; heart rate, (f$_h$) is 110/minutes.
One week later, a load of 75 watts (performed without
β-blockers) is stopped after 2 minutes 15 owing to angina,
a heart rate of 114/minute being achieved; during recovery,
ST segment elevation and severe ventricular arrhythmia
occur. More severe electrocardiographic ischaemia for
a same of lower myocardial oxygen demand (practically
same heart rate on exercise, lower workload on shorter
working time) suggests coronary spasm.

4.   Arrhythmias on Exercise

     Cardiac arrhythmias are extremely frequent at rest as well
as during exercise, even in apparently healthy subjects, which has
been confirmed by Holter monitor electrocardiography. Their
precise clinical and diagnostic significance is not well known
yet but it is true that they may have dramatic consequences in a
limited number of cases, most often in patients with coronary
disease.

     We studied (3) the incidence and types of arrhythmias
observed during exercise testing of 1628 subjects. Among them,
736 were apparently healthy and had a normal exercise test, 182
had coronary insufficiency demonstrated angiographically or by a
positive ECG response to exercise, 710 had previously a
myocardial infarction diagnosed by a typical Q wave or by
significant enzymatic changes. In all cases, the ECG was
recorded continuously during 5 minutes at rest, during a
progressive exercise test and during at least the first 5 minutes
of the recovery period.

     Arrhythmias were observed in 37% of apparently healthy subjects,
48% of coronary patients without myocardial necrosis and 61% of
patients with previous myocardial infarction. The difference is
statistically significant between the first and the two other
groups. A difference was also found for supraventricular and
ventricular isolated premature beats but it is only statistically
significant for the group with previous myocardial infarction;
it is significant for both groups of coronary patients as far as
severe ventricular premature beats are concerned (i.e. bigeminism,
multifocal ectopy or runs of premature beats) : 7% in healthy
subjects, 13% in coronary patients without myocardial necrosis,
22% in patients with myocardial infarction. A difference was
also observed for ventricular premature beats on exercise, rest
being not taken into consideration; however it is only statistically
significant for the group with previous myocardial infarction.

     Ventricular premature beats, which are by far the more
frequent, were studied for several correlations:

     In patients with previous myocardial infarction, ventricular
premature beats at rest and during exercise, or during exercise
only, showed no relationship with ST segment changes on effort
(the latter were classified into four categories: no ST changes,
JST depression with slowly upsloping ST segment or ST depression
less than .1 mV, significant horizontal ST depression of at
least .1 mV, ST segment elevation of at least .1 mV compared to
rest). The same lack of relationship exists for casual (<5/mn)
or severe premature ventricular beats.

Among patients who had an angiogram, ventricular ectopy
showed no relationship with the number of coronary vessels
significantly altered (>70% stenosis). It seems, however, that
3-vessel lesions produce more ventricular premature beats than
single- or 2-vessel lesions when no myocardial infarction is
present and that in cases with myocardial infarction ventricular
ectopy is more frequent already at rest, probably owing to the
presence of a myocardial scar rather than to the coronary
alterations.

In healthy subjects, occasional ore repetitive ventricular
premature beats on exercise show a linear relationship with
heart rate and arterial blood pressure; only the relationship
between severe ectopy and heart rate is not statistically
significant. Moreover, ventricular premature beats on exercise
increase with systolic blood pressure within the different
classes of heart rate. In patients with myocardial infarction,
however, such a correlation is not found, ventricular premature
beats being merely more frequent beyond a systolic pressure of
150mm Hg.

SUMMARY

a) Arrhythmias at rest and on effort are more frequent
    in coronary patients than in healthy subjects but
    ventricular ectopy shows relationship neither with
    exercise-induced ST segment changes nor with the extension
    of coronary lesions; after myocardial infarction, the
    occurence of ventricular premature beats seems to be
    essentially due to the cardiac scar;

b) in healthy subjects, ventricular ectopy seems to be more
    related to the heart work level;

c) until now, information is lacking concerning the remote
    prognosis of resting and exercise-induced ventricular
    arrhythmias occuring in healthy subjects and in patients
    with coronary heart disease.

References

1. E. A. Amsterdam, J. H. Wilmore and A. N. DeMaria. Exercise
    in cardiovascular health and disease, pp.188-208, Yorke
    Medical Books, New York (1977).
2. B. Demaret, R. Messin, Ph. Salhadin, P. Block et van E. Thiel.
    Difficultés d'exécution et d'interprétation de l'épreuve
    d'effort chez la femme. In: "Les épreuves d'effort.
    Colloque d'Ambarès, juin 1977", pp.7-13. J.P. Broustet, H.
    Bricaud et H. Denolin éds. Expansion Scientifique, Paris
    (1978).

3. B. Demaret, R. Messin, and Ph. Salhadin. Incidence and
    significance of exercise-induced arrhythmias in healthy
    subjects and in patients with coronary heart disease
    (1978).

4. G. Dereume et B. Demaret. Modifications électrocardiographiques
    liées à un syndrome de Wolff-Parkinson-White intermittent
    au cours d'une épreuve d'effort (To be published).

5. R. Messin. The practice and limitation factors of ergometric
    tests. In: "Ergebnisse der Ergometrie", pp. 85-90. H.
    Mellerowicz, E. Jockl and G. Hansen eds. Perimed Verlag Dr.
    med. D. Straube, Erlangen, (1975).

6. Org. Mond. Sante. Registres de l'infarctus du myocarde.
    Résultats d'une étude coopérative internationale de l'OMS,
    coordonnée par le Bureau Régional de l'Europe, p.61.
    La Santé Publique en Europe, p.61. La Santé Publique en
    Europe 5, Copenhague, (1977).

7. Ph. Salhadin, M. Lebedelle, van E. Thiel, B. Demaret, P.
    Vandermoten et H. Denolin. L'apparition à l'effort de
    l'image de lésion sous-épicardique en l'absence de signes
    de nécrose myocardique. Etude clinique, électrocardiographique
    et coronarographique de 10 cas. Acta Cardiol. (Brux.)
    6:401-422, (1977).

VALUE OF EXERCISE TESTING ON ANGINA PECTORIS FOR PREDICTION OF LIFE EXPECTANCY, LEFT VENTRICULAR FUNCTION AND CORONARY LESIONS

J.P. Broustet, J.F. Cherrier, and P. Guern

Département des épreuves d'effort et Service
de Cardiologie A
Hopital Cardiologique du Haut Leveque
33604 - Pessac, France

Although many studies, especially the Framingham study (1), have demonstrated the statistical severity of coronary heart disease (CHD) prognosis, appraisal of individual life expectancy has been a challenge for a long time, before the onset of clinically obvious circulatory failure. The "30 seconds of 30 years" as expressed by Gallavardin sixty years ago indicate what was the range of standard deviation for a clever observer of the natural history of CHD.

For a long time exercise training (ET) as performed by Master test has made possible the diagnosis and helped to identify the ischemic byt asymptomatic patients.

Indeed three facts improved the prognosis value of ET:

First of all the correlations with coronary angiography (CA). In spite of some controversies due to a too rigid and rough definition of both ischemia and "positive" CA, concordance is sufficient enough (80 to 90%) to ensure a respective validation of these two investigations and to ensure a correct prognosis value to these investigations.

Secondly the obsolete Master Test was replaced by maximal ET or symptom limited ET (SLET) more precise and more safe.

Thirdly the ECG criteria are no longer the only to be studied: the circulatory parameters, the exercise capacity data provide more and more valuable informations.

The main questions which deal with prognosis value of ET
are the following:

1°)   In asymptomatic patients what is predictive value of
       negative or positive ET for future occurrence of coronary
       event (angina, infarction, sudden death)?

2°)   In coronary patient does ET still have a prognosis
       value that ET may provide information concerning life
       expectancy: the attempt to answer this second question
       used two ways.

       a)   by means of long term follow up in coronary
             patients after the first exercise test: this approach
             is rather new and will provide data in the near
             future.

       b)   by means of comparisons with angiographic and
             hemodynamic ventriculographic data. It is then
             necessary to quantify with accuracy ET and CA data
             and to look for correlations. This last approach
             relies on data in literature concerning angiographic
             results (studies of Cleveland Clinic for example).

PREDICTIVE VALUE OF EXERCISE TEST IN ASYMPTOMATIC PATIENTS

It is well established that an ischemic S-T segment
depression (S-T↓) defined as S-T↓⩾ 1 mm is an indication or
elevated risk of further coronary event. Robb (2) in life
insurance subcriptors pointed out that post exercise S-T↓⩾ of 1 mm
implies 4.3 more risks that in normals. If S-T↓ is ⩾ 2 mm the
risk reaches 15.8 by regard to normal post exercise S-T segment.

Beard (3) performed Master test in asymptomatic population
8% were considered as positive: 60% of these positive had a
coronary event within the following 30 months.

Doyle and Kinch (4) exercised 2003 asymptomatic patients
and repeated ET in those who had S-T↓ or exercise induced left
bundle branch block : within 5 years, 85% of the patients
belonging to this group developed a coronary event. Moreover the
authors provided information concerning sensitivity and specificity.
Among 264 patients having coronary event during follow up only
75 had an abnormal first ET and represented 85% of positive ET.
Conversely 189 patients developed further coronary event in spite
of negative ET. Thus the predictive value was weak. Indeed these
ET were not maximal. But finally the probability to NOT HAVE
coronary event within the next five years was 13.6% in patients
with positive ET versus 98.5% in those with negative ET.

Many data reinforced these results: Kattus (5) in 314 normal clerks performing a near maximal ET on treadmill found 30 S-T↘ during exercise or recovery without angina. There was a strong correlation with risks factors (hypertension, cigarettes, cholesterol). Within 2.5 next years, among these 30 patients occurred : 3 coronary deaths, 4 infarctions, 2 angina pectoris. In negative ET group, there was no coronary event during the same period.

In the "7 countries study" Blackburn (6) demonstrated that a post exercise S-T↘ indicates 3 times more coronary risks than junctional depression or negativation of T waves.

In air force or civil pilots maximal ET are periodically performed and when S-T↘ is observed, CA is performed even in asymptomatic patients. Froelicher (7) followed 1390 asymptomatic men (mean age: 38 ± 8 years) for 6.3 years after initial maximal ET: among this cohort 710 had normal data and no risk factor: only 7 had coronary event during the follow up period, 17 patients had ischemic S-T↘ and did not have coronary event during the follow up period. 123 had hypertension: 5 had a positive stress test. Among them 3 had coronary event. It is well known now that in normals the false positive rate is too high as demonstrated by Erickssen in Oslo (31). Froelicher (7) systematically performed CA in 76 asymptomatic patients with normal resting ECG and exercise induced S-T↘

47% had normal coronary angiogram

9% had lesion < 50% of diameter of vessels

43% had stenosis >50%

Bruce (8) studied 1820 formosans 40 to 59 years old for seven years after maximal ET. Only 220 developed a coronary event (less than 2%/years).

The total incidence of coronary event was:

2.3% in subject with normal S-T

5.7% in those with S-T↘≥ 1 mm

11.9% in hypertension

25% in hypertension + S-T↘

Bruce again (9) in "Seattle Heart Watch" followed for 24.6 months 3132 normal men (mean age: 45 years) after maximal ET on treadmill.

Total annual incidence of coronary event was 1.5/1000, the rate was 0.6/1000 when S-T↓ was <1 mm versus, 8.9/1000 when S-T↓ ≥ 1 mm.

Wilhemsen (10) studied 803 normal men born in 1913. They carried out ET at the time of entrance into study. After 8 years, 49 infarction occurred of which 20 were fatal: the predictive value of S-T↓ was 3/1. Indeed 50% of future infarction had normal exercise test but most of them had chronotropic incompetence and elevation of respiratory frequency.

Indeed exercise induced hemodynamic abnormalities may be observed a part from S-T segment variations and seem to have heavy significance,Ellestad (11) performed maximal ET in 1067 patients: S-T↓ did not appear.

Among 85 who did not reach a heart rate of 95% of the standard deviation for age coronary event occurred with anormal incidence of 150/1000 the same as in those with 4 mm S-T↓ ! Conversely patients with normal maximal heart rate had a year incidence of 1.7/1000 only.

The same author (12) showed that the delay of onset of S-T has a stronger predictive value than the amplitude of S-T↓ . Conversely the delay for recovery of resting S-T after S-T↓ is not a good predictor.

The high significance of poor elevation of HR during exercise is well explained by the close relationship between exercise coronary output or myocardial oxygen consumption on one hand and heart rate (r = 0.82) or double product heart rate x systolic blood pressure (r = 0.88) on the other hand (13).

Thus a patient who reaches a high heart rate in spite of huge S-T has probably a local deficit in coronary perfusion associated to a good total coronary output. When the critical heart rate is low there is probably both diffuse coronary stenosis and poor contractility.

Kramer (14) found 28 negative ET in a group of patients with severe coronary lesions: 23 among these 28 patients had severe hypokinesia or akinesia of left ventricle. Thus the aptitude to depress S-T segment does imply a good parietal thickness of contractile but ischemic myocardium.

PREDICTIVE VALUE OF EXERCISE TEST IN CORONARY PATIENTS

After myocardial infarction S-T↓ has a bad prognosis. It is obvious that ischemia in area else than the infarcted area predict two or triple vessel disease. Exercise induced S-T↓ is very rare in a lead where significant Q wave is present (32).

Schaeffer (15) found 25 negative and 7 positive ET after infarction in 32 patients.

One year later amond these 7 patients, three had angina, one died suddenly, one had new infarction versus one sudden death, among the 25 negative tests.

Predictive value of exercise capacity. The relationship between left ventricular performance and exercise capacity are strong and help to understand the proeminent prevalence of exercise capacity in prognosis of angina pectoris.

Margolis (16) found a strong correlation between life expectancy at two years and exercise test duration using Bruce protocole (Table 1).

Conversely in this group neither the extent of coronary disease nor amplitude of S-T↘ or left ventriculography data allowed such a discrimination. These data are actually very important when one has to decide indication for coronary by pass in patients who are associated with significant stenosis and excellent exercise capacity.

Ellestad (8) performed maximal symptom limited ET in patients referred for chest pain.

Among those having S-T↘> 1.5 mm the year incidence of mortality was: 9.5% versus, 1.7% in those with S-T↘ <0.5mm. Indeed among those with S-T↘ >1.5mm, the year incidence was 15% when S-T ↘ appeared at low exercise level (≥ 4 mets) which year incidence was only 4% when S-T occurred at 8 mets.

TABLE I

% Survival After Two Years and Numbers of Stages Achieved

	Stages			
	I	II	III	IV
Medically treated N = 378	54%			99%
By passed N = 323	82%			98%

Moreover amplitude of S-T↓ from 1.5 to 4 mm had no predictive value!

CORRELATIONS BETWEEN EXERCISE TEST DATA AND ANGIOGRAPHIC AND HEMODYNAMIC DATA

Their interest is growing since, there are many data on predictive value of number, topography of coronary stenosis, and left ventricular performance as appreciated from kinetics or ejection fraction determination.

Coronary lesions and risks of sudden death. Bruschke (17) reported the rate of death after one and five years following the number of coronary vessels with stenosis - 50%. (Table II).

A very narrow stenosis had a worst future than a thrombosis as confirmed by Kattus (18). He reported a year incidence of death of 6% in patients with thrmobose and collateral against 10.6% in patients with two stenosis.

Webster (18) eliminated coronary patients with impairment of left ventricular function; in the remaining he studied the prognosis of proximal stenosis (Table III).

TABLE II

	DEATH RATE %	
	1 year	5 years
No. of involved vessels		
One vessel	2.92	14.6
Two vessels	7.56	37.8
Three vessels	10.76	53.8
Left main trunk	11.36	56.8

TABLE III

	DEATH RATE %	
	1 year	6 years
No. of involved vessels		
One vessel (no.178)	4	25.5
Two vessels (no.177)	7	41.5
Three vessels (no.114	10.5	63
Left main trunk (no.21)	11.8	71

Moreover, data concerning the stenosed vessels are important to precise (Table IV).

Does exercise test help to predict number and topography of lesions and thus the prognosis?

Left main trunk lesions are often predicted from ET data: in such patients Cohen and Gorlin (20) using Master test in spite of its poor sensitivity found that 34 pts among 48 had S-T↓ > 2mm. In six patients S-T↓ ranged between 1 and 2 millimeters. Seven patients did not demonstrate S-T changes. Indeed among the 7 pts with no S-T↓ , 6 had a critical heart rate <110/mm.

In our center, we studied 276 patients (mean age 53 years ±9) suffering angina or having recently spontaneous angina and having one or more stenosis over 50% on one or several coronary arteries.

Every patient had maximal or symptom limited exercise test; maximal ET was defined by an exercise rate ⩾220-age. Some patients did not reach this value for they stopped before for leg pain or important dyspnea and or fatigue. The remaining patients were interrupted only when frank anginal pain appeared. Isolated S-T↓ whatever its amplitude was never a criteria for cessation of test except when frequent ventricular premature beats occurred.

TABLE IV

		DEATH RATE %	
		1 year	6 years
One vessel	right C.Art	2.3	14
	left ant.desc.	4.1	24.6
	circumflex	4.2	25
Two vessels	right cor. + circumflex	5.9	35.4
	left ant.desc + circumflex	7.8	47
	right cor. art + left ant. desc.	6.8	41

70 patients had single vessel disease, 72 double vessel disease, 104 triple vessel disease; 30 had left main trunk disease usually associated to stenosis involving other arteries.

Thus critical heart rate was diminished following the number of involved vessels but not into discriminant range.

Critical or maximal systolic blood pressure (CSBP)TABLE V(a),(b). The same was true for CSBP and for the double product (HR x CSBP) (Table VI).

Thus these circulatory parameters are not discriminant enough to prodict the number of narrowed vessels. Indeed when they are at high levels a single vessel disease remains predictable. Conversely if the double product is below 2000 Hg/ cm/min multivessel disease is predictable.

TABLE V(a)

Critical heart rate (CHR)

	1 v. (70)	2 v. (72)	3 v. (104)	Left main trunk (30)	Normals
"Critical heart rate"	138 ± 25	+133 − 26	+130 − 22	125 ± 28	165 ± 10

TABLE V(b)

"Critical" Systolic Blood Pressure (CBS)

	1 v. (70)	2 v. (72)	3 v. (104)	Tr g (30)
S BP (mmHg)	+185 − 29	185 ± 29	168 ± 33	±36

TABLE VI

"Critical" Values of Double Product (HR x SBP)

	1 v. (70)	2 v. (72)	3 v. (104)	Tr g (30)	Normals
HR x SBP (cmHg/min	2553	2460	2288	2100	3500

Exercise Capacity. Exercise capacity was in any way the most predictive parameter (Table VII).

TABLE VII

Total Work (Kpm)

	1 v.	2 v.	3 v.	Left main trunk	Normals
Total work (Kpm)	4718 ±2549	4360 ±2487	3076 ±2129	2671 ±1596	6300 to 11340
Correspondance in watts in 30 W/3 min increment protocole	120 W 2min 5	120 W 1min15	90 W 2min 45	90 W 2min	150 W 1 min 180 W 3 min

The single vessel patients had an exercise capacity near of twice the capacity of left main trunk. Unfortunately the great standard deviation did not allow a high discriminant value but it is obvious that the association of low levels for critical HR, SBP, and poor exercise capacity carries a strong risk of multivessel disease, especially if coupled with S-T↓ amplitude. Multivariate analysis is in progression but up to now, we are not able to present data.

S-T segment depression (Table VIII). There was a good relationship with the number of narrowed vessels in spite of many infarcted patients (47) in the group of triple vessel disease.

TABLE VIII

Amplitude of S-T segment depression
in CM5 lead
after exclusion of 6 LBB blocks

	1 v. (70)	2 v. (72)	3 v. (104)	Left main trunk (28)
S-T (mm)	1.5 ±0.8	1.91 ±1.7	2.29 ±1.42	3.34 ±1.6

Predictive value of symptom limited exercise test for life
expectancy was studied essentially in the triple vessel disease
group.

Patients were followed for a mean duration of 26 months
±12 months, 16 died from coronary death 88 survived, 37 were by
passed with no hospital or further death.

Predictive value of exercise capacity was better for life
expectancy than to separate the number of narrowed vessels
(Table IX).

Thus the exercise capacity in survivors was almost twice
more than in dead patients. The mean value of resting ejection
fraction as calculated from left ventricule angiographic data was
0.65 in survivors, 0.52 in non survivors. Indeed there was a
poor linear correlation coefficient between these two parameters.

Conversely the amplitude of S-T↓ was not significantly different
between survivors and non survivors. While the time of onset of
S-T↓ (S-T≥1mm regarding the resting values) was very discriminant
(Table X).

These data have been well supported by further clinical
observations and follow up of these patients.

On the other hand among the patients with triple vessels
disease, a score of coronary lesions was not of help for prediction
of life expectancy. This score relied on number, proximal or
distal situation of stenosis, degree of narrowing, absence or
presence of collateral, quality of distal bed.

TABLE IX

Triple vessel disease (104 patients)
mean follow up : 26 months

	Total Work : Kpm
All patients (104)	3076 ± 2152
Cardiac death (16)	2179 ± 1101
By passed (37)	2684 ± 1913
Unoperated and alive (51)	3484 ± 2251

TABLE X

Triple vessel disease
time of onset of S-T depression
work achieved when S-T↓ has increased of 1 mm

	Dead (16)	Alive (88)
Work (Kpm)	895 ±625	1529 ± 963 $p<0.005$

Table XI show the poor difference in alive and dead patients.

TABLE XI

Coronary lesion scores

	1 v. (70)	2 v. (72)	3 v. (104)
Score	4.3 ⁺1.3	8.29 ⁺1.81	12.9 ± 2

TABLE IX (continued)

Triple vessel disease

	Dead (16)	Alive (88)	
Score	13.5 ±2	12.5 ±1.9	(NS)

There is more and more reliable data in literature reporting good global correlation between exercise test data and coronary lesions:

Romhilt (21) compared the extent of lesions by means of Friesinger index with the non electrocardiographic exercise data in 40 patients (Table XII).

Thus even when pain is lacking, if they are gathered: low critical HR, low increase in SBP, huge S-T↓ , low exercise capacity, the probability of severe diffuse stenosis or of left main trunk is strong enough to lead to coronary angiogram.

TABLE XII

Relationship between non electrocardiographic
data and coronary score in
40 patients with angina

	r value for Friesinger index	P value
Exercise duration (ED)	0.55	0.001
Maximal heart rate (MHR)	0.62 (Infarction:0.77)	"
Increase in heart rate	0.64 (Infarction:0.71)	" "
Product (ED x MHR)	0.60	"
VO2 max S.L.	0.47	"

In our 104 patients with angina pectoris and triple vessel
disease:

3 patients had maximal and normal exercise tests for exercise
capacity, circulatory adaptation, S-T segment; one of three had
typical anginal pain at the end of test. May be these patients
could have positive exercise test if they have been started at
their maximal level.

7 patients had no S-T segment changes during exercise:

5 had large anterior infarction

1 had left bundle branch block

1 has ventricular premature beats
but in these seven cases, the critical heart rate was 130/min
and the maximal load 90 watts for 1.5 minute in left main trunks.

These examples stress on the fact that S-T segment changes
are not the only interesting end point of exercise test. The
whole feature of all parameters has to be considered, for example
changes in blood pressure must be carefully studied: thus Thompson
(22) found in twelve patients a decrease in blood pressure during
exercise (mean value: -3.3 mmHg) at the onset of anginal pain. No
patients could reach a HR of 150/min. None had a rest sign or
symptoms of cardiac failure but one had ejection fraction of
LV < 0.45.

Two on 10 patients died suddenly before coronary angiogram.

10/10 had a stenosis ≥ 75% on left anterior descending artery
and another trunk.

5/10 had triple vessel disease

3/10 had left main trunk stenosis

5/10 could be by passed. None of them had exercise induced
hypotension after surgery.

Timmis (23) observed 27 patients with significant stenosis
of left main trunk or both circumflex and left anterior descending.

16 had no exercise induced S-T segment changes

3 had a critical heart rate < 110 BPM

7 are below 85% of maximal HR

6 reach 85%

Exercise testing and left ventricular kinetics. Bungraaf (24) emphasized that with identical coronary lesion, the risk of death in the further 5 years has a considerable range following the left ventricular kinetics (Table XIII).

TABLE XIII

Left ventricular kinetics

% Death Rate at 5 Years

	Normal Kinetics	Local Alteration	Diffuse Alteration
1 v.	7%	15%	60%
3 v.	35%	50%	88%

Bruschke (25) provided same range of information (Table XIV): whatever the number of involved vessels, he reported the following data:-

TABLE XIV

	% Death	
	At One Year	At Five Years
Normal kinetics	5	25
Local hypokinesia	6.2	31
Local dyskinesia and normal kinetics of the rest of LV	9.2	46
Local dyskinesia and diffuse hypokinesia	12.8	64
Diffuse hypokinesia	14.2	71

Does exercise test allow to predict left ventricular kinetics?

Until now the answer is not frankly affirmative. It is obvious that after infarction, the lead facing the area of necrosis even after disappearance of Q wave, will exhibit S-T segment elevation, sometimes very important always corresponding to akinetic, hypokinetic or dyskinetic areas at left ventriculography. But this last investigation is usually done at rest, thus

paroxystic dyskinesia is only probable but unproven. In the absence
of previous history of myocardial infarction, exercise induced
S-T elevation is very rare, may be enhanced by beta-blockade
therapy and correspond to sudden transmural ischemia with
transitory dyskinesia : in such conditions the relation from
Prinzmetal variant is unclear : usually severe lesions are present
(26).

Indeed S-T↓ remains a valuable indicator of coronary lesions
Bartel (27) shown that the percentage of positive test for S-T↓
was:

40% in single vessel disease

66% in double vessel disease

76% in triple vessel disease

McHenry (28) using computerized index of S-T slope and S-T
depression as an index for ischemia reported similar results
(Table XV).

TABLE XV

No. of involved vessels	Ischemic index value (S-T slope and S-T depression)	
	End of the test	Recovery
1 (35 pts)	-0.76	+0.17
2 (64 pts)	-1.42	-0.35
3 (45 pts)	-1.50	-0.63

These data are reliable but once again leave to much
variations when dealing with individual patient.

Prognosis value of exercise induced arrythmias (EIA). It is
necessary to observe their frequency, and their morphology: some
isolated VPB occurring at the very onset of exercise or at the
end of maximal exercise test will not have the same meaning as
polymorph VBP increasing as HR, bouts of ventricular tachycardia.

Simoons (29), Blackburn (6) do not give to exercise induced VBP a strong predictive value concerning sudden death. Indeed Nead (30) stressed their importance in coronary patients submitted to physical training:

15 cardiac arrest (CA) occurred between 1968 and 1975 in regularly trained patients (1 CA for 6,000 hour/patients of supervised training).

12 among 15 had suffered previous myocardial infarction.

The mean duration of training was 18 months.

10 among 15 had many VPB on control exercise test.

4 had a decrease in SBP at the last stage of exercise test.

13 survived their cardiac arrest.

2/15 received both digitalis and diuretics.

McHenry (33) pointed out that the level of heart rate at the time of onset of VBP is important to check in patients who had VBP under 130 BPM the proportion of coronary patient was high. By means of the Rowe index, he found out a correlation between the frequency of VBP and the extension of coronary lesions.

The reproducibility of exercise induced VBP remains statistically questionable. In our experience a little number of coronary patients will have VBP at every exercise test while most of them will not have reproducible VBP.

Finally there is a gap between this large amount of statistical data and the individual patient problem. Is he in the 20% who will not die before seven or ten years? Or conversely does he belong to the "2% group"?

Multivariate analysis may help a more comprehensive and at the same time personnalized approach but it must itself rely on a perfect collect of data at the time of exercise test and during prolonged follow up of large series. These studies are very difficult to carry out by one single group and loose a big part of their accuracy when they are cooperative.

The upper data lead to the following and provisory statements.

1) the primary aim of clinician is to identify ischemia and to try to quantify it in terms of exercise capacity, heart rate and blood pressure elevation, S-T segment changes whatever the formulae used.

2) Then being aware of the strong relationship between coronary lesions, vital prognosis, left ventricular function and data he must decide if a coronary angiogram is useful, if surgery appears necessary.

The wrong way being to perform first coronary angiogram and then to go back to exercise test to decide if there are false positive or for negative data or to try to justify and a prior indication for surgery.

3) At the individual level, when there is no scientific or safety purpose it is not useful to perform maximal exercise in asymptomatic patients. This procedure may lead to false positive results.

References

1. W. B. Kannel, B. Feinlet. Natural history of angina pectoris in the Framingham study. Prognosis and survival. Amer. J. Cardiol. 29:154 (1972)
2. G. P. Robb, H. H. Marks. Post exercise electrocardiogram in arteriosclerotic heart disease. J.A.M.A., 200:918 (1967).
3. E. F. Beard, E. Garcia, G. E. Burke, W. E. Daar. Post exercise electrocardiogram in screening for latent ischemic heart disease. Dis Chest, 56:405 (1969).
4. J. T. Doyle, S. W. Kinch. Prognosis of an abnormal electro-cardiographic stress test. Circ. 41:545 (1970).
5. A. A. Kattus, C. R. Jorgensen, R. E. Worden, A. N. Alvaro. S-T segment depression with near maximal exercise in detection of pre-clinical coronary heart disease. Circulation 44:585 (1971).
6. H. Blackburn, H. L. Taylor, A. Keys. The electrocardiogram in prediction of five year coronary heart disease incidence among men aged forty through to fifty nine. Coronary heart disease in seven countries. Circulation 41, suppl. 1:1 154 (1970).
7. V. Froelicher, Mary N. M. Thomas, C. S. Pillow, M. C. Lancaster. Epidemiologic study of asymptomatic men screen by maximal treadmill testing for latent coronary artery disease. Am.J. of Card. 34:770 (1974).
8. R. A. Bruce, Y. Pao, N. Ting, Y. Chiang, S. T. Chiang, E. R. Alexander, R. Beasley, L. D. Fisher. Seven year follow up of cardiovascular study and maximal exercise testing of chinese men. Circulation, 51:890 (1975).
9. R. A. Bruce, B. S. Chinn, M. B. Irving, T. De Roven. Clinical and exercise predictors of coronary heart disease mortality in men. Abstract 679: 7ème Congrés Europeen de Cardiologie - Ambsterdam Juin 76.

10. L. Wilhelmsen. Exercise tests in screening for heart
    disease. Abstract 678 : 7ème Congrés Européen de Cardiologie
    - Amsterdam Juin 76.

11. M. H. Ellestad, M. F. C. Wan. Predictive implications of
    stress testing follow up of 2700 subjects after maximum
    treadmill stress testing. Circulation 51:363 (1975).

12. M. H. Ellestad. Stress testing. Principles and practice
    1 vol. F. A. Davis - Philadelphia 1975.

13. R. R. Nelson, F. L. Gobel, C. R. Jorgensen, K. Wang, Y. Wang,
    H. L. Taylor. Hemodynamic predictors of myocardial oxygen
    consumption during static and dynamic exercise. Circulation
    50:1179 (1974).

14. N. E. Kramer, A. Susmano, M. S. Rosenberg, R. B. Shekell.
    Left ventricular dysfunction and false negative response to
    treadmill exercise test. Circulation 51-52:Suppl.II,
    47 Abstract 179 (1975).

15. C. W. Schaeffer, R. G. Daly, S. C. Smith. Maximal treadmill
    exercise testing in the management of the post myocardial
    infarction patient. Chest 68:20 (1975).

16. J. R. Margolis. Treadmill stage as a predictor of medical
    surgical survival in coronary disease.

17. A. V. G. Bruschke, W. L. Proudfit, F. M. Sones. Progress
    study of 590 consecutive non surgical cases of coronary
    disease followed 5-9 years. I - Arteriographic correlations.
    Circulation, 47:1147 (1973).

18. A. A. Kattus. Relation of coronary events to spasm of
    coronary arteris, precariousness of obstructive lesions and
    of collaterals chawed in current topics in coronary research.
    Advances in Experimental Medicine and Biology Vol.39
    Bloor and Olsson ed., Plenum Press, London 1973.

19. J. S. Webster, C. Moberg, G. Rincon. Natural history of
    severe proximal coronary artery disease as documented by
    coronary cineangiography. Amer. J. Cardiol., 33:195 (1974).

20. M. V. Cohen, R. Gorlin. Main left coronary areery disease
    clinical experience from 1964-1974. Circulation, 52:275
    (1975).

21. D. Romhilt, E. McCall, I. Grais, H. Spitz, J. Holmes, R.
    Adolph. Correlation of submaximal graded treadmill exercise
    test with severity of coronary artery disease on coronary
    angiography. Circulation, Suppl. IV 47:208 Abstract No.827
    (1973).

22. P. D. Thompson, M. H. Kelemen. A reliable and easily
    elicited of critical coronary narrowing. Circulation,
    49-50: Suppl. III 9 (1974).

23. G. Timmis, S. Gordon, R. Ramos, V. Gangadharan, W. Beaumont.
    The failure of submaximal stress testing to identify
    "critical" left coronary artery (LCA) disease. Circulation
    Suppl. II 51-52: LL 47 Abstract 178 (1975).

24. G. W. Burggraf, J. O. Parker. Prognosis in coronary artery
    disease : angiographic, hemodynamic, and clinical factors.
    Circulation, 51:147 (1975).
25. A. V. G. Bruschke, W. L. Proudfit, F. M. Sones. Progress study
    of 590 consecutive non surgical cases of coronary disease
    followed 5-9 years. II - Ventriculographic and other
    correlations. Circulation, 47:1154 (1973).
26. N. J. Fortuin, C. G. Fiesinger. Exercise induced S-T segment
    elevation. Clinical, electrocardiographic and arteriographic
    study in twelve patients. Amer. J. Med. 49:459 (1970).
27. A. G. Bartel, V. S. Behar, R. H. Peter, S. E. Orgain, Y. Kong.
    Graded exercise stress tests in angiographically documented
    coronary artery disease. Circulation, 49:Fev. (1974).
28. P. L. McHenry, S. N. Morris. Prediction of severity of
    coronary disease by exercise S-T segment response. Circulation
    Suppl. II 51-52:676 Abstract 175 (1975).
29. M. L. Simoons, J. J. R. Bonnier, J. Pool. Prediction of
    sudden death from exercise ECG. Abstract 629 - 7ème Congrés
    Europeén de Cardiologie - Amsterdam Juin 1976.
30. W. F. Nead, H. R. Pyfer, J. C. Trombold, R. C. Frederick.
    Successful resuscitation of two near simultaneous cases of
    cardiac with a review of fifteen cases occuring during
    supervised exercise. Circulation, 53:187 (1976).
31. R. Haiat, J. P. Broustet. L'électrocardiogramme d'effort après
    la phase aiguë de l'infarctus du myocarde : analyse de 100 cas.
    Nouvelle Presse Médicale, 5, No 12, 775, (1976).
32. P. L. McHenry, S. N. Morris, M. Kavalier, J. W. Jordan.
    Comparative study of exercise induced ventricular arrythmias
    in normal subjects and patients with documented coronary
    artery disease. Am. J. Cardiol., 37:609 (1976).

FREQUENCY OF VENTRICULAR ECTOPIC ACTIVITY RECORDED DURING

EXERCISE STRESS TEST AND CONTINUOUS HOLTER MONITORING

Jan J. Kellermann, E. Ben-Ari, and N. Lederman

Cardiac Evaluation and Rehabilitation Institute
Chaim Sheba Medical Center and Tel Aviv University
Medical School
Tel Hashomer
Israel

INTRODUCTION

Of late, more studies are available comparing exercise testing
and Holter monitoring, especially in relation to the detection
of arrhythmias. All over the world big efforts are being made to
combat sudden death and in the framework of these undertakings the
early detection of arrhythmias has naturally gained increasing
importance.

All these studies are still in a preliminary stage. But it
seems to us that the accumulation of data and especially a long
term follow up may eventually assist in reaching a conclusion as
to which preventive measures should be undertaken in order to
decrease the incidence of sudden death, especially in middle aged
men.

This paper is based on two study reports:

The first study, comprising 75 patients after transmural
myocardial infarction who are undergoing a prolonged continuous
rehabilitation program, and the second study, comprising additional
93 rehabilitated coronary patients divided into symptomatic
asymptomatic groups. The aim of our study was to find out whether
or not the appearance and frequency of VEA during exercise stress
testing, based on a multistage gradual increment of work loads,
compared to 24 hours Holter monitoring, shows differences. It was
our intention to determine the effect of the heart rate frequency
on appearance of VEA and whether or not psychosocial stimuli of

daily life activities without relation to heart rate frequencies have impact on the electrical instability of the heart.

STUDY I (13)

Material

75 patients with coronary heart disease (with and without angina pectoris),mean age 52.7 years $\pm$ 7,6 years undergoing continuous supervised rehabilitation in the mean of 4,1 years were included in this study. 78.3% of these patients had a single transmural infarction and 21.7% a subendocardial infarction. The mean time since the acute onset was 6,3 years. 51.3% complained of angina pectoris. A number of patients with angina pectoris received nitrites and beta-blocking drugs, but treatment was stopped 48 hours prior to the exercise test and on the day of the recording.

Methods

a)   All patients underwent repeated multistage discontinuous ergometric tests. After a detailed history in which special attention is given to the patient's physical activities, a physical examination, electrocardiogram and radiogram of the chest are obtained. If there are no signs of acute cardiac insufficiency, severe multifocal ventricular arrhythmia, if the diastolic blood pressure is not above 115 mm.Hg. and the patient is not suffering from intractable angina pectoris, an ergometric or spiroergometric test is performed to determine submaximal (80%-85% of maximal heart rate) physical working capacity (PWC). (1, 2, 3).

b)   Holter Avionics recorders 445 and Electrocardioscanner 660 have been used for recording and replay. Together 1800 recording hours were monitored. Because of the fact that the most common activities recorded were driving, exercise training, daily work, leisure time (TV), sex and sleep, we have concentrated only on the collection of data of these activities. Ventricular ectopic activity (VEA) recorded during exercise stress testing was compared to VEA recorded at the various aforementioned activities.

     The heart rate (HR) during the various activities was determined by measuring the frequency at different time intervals of the specific activity. If VEA occured, the frequency of the regular sinus complexes close to VEA was determined also. The mean values were calculated from several frequence measurements of the same activity.

c)   Statistical assessment was done by means of the analysis of variance for a single factor with repeated measures on the

same elements and the analysis of variance for the mean values
of a parameter obtained in 3 different situations. For the
purpose of statistical analysis, data of 55 out of the 75
patients were used, because only patients where at least 3
situations were recorded - such as exercise test, driving and
daily work were chosed.

RESULTS

1.   Submaximal Ergometric Test (4)

The submaximal heart rate (HR) obtained in the 75 patients
was 131.9 $\pm$ 20 beats/min. (b/m). The patients with angina
pectoris (A.P.) (38 patients) had a mean exercise HR of
130 b/m and the group without A.P. (36 patients) a mean HR of
138 b/m. (One patient with myocardial infarction by history,
was excluded from further assessments). The mean physical work
capacity (PWC) for the angina group was 85.8 Watt which
represents 68% of the norm of healthy male individuals as
standardized at our institute according to age. The group
without A.P. had a mean PWC of 95 Watt which represents 76%
of the norm. The double product was 21,900 for the angina
group and 24,300 for the non-angina group. These results
point to the fact that the physical capabilities of both
groups were more than satisfactory and demonstrate a fairly
high PWC.

2.   Heart Rate (Holter Recording)

a)   During driving under heavy traffic conditons of at least
      45-50 minutes duration, in 66 out of the 75 patients,
      the mean HR recorded was 106 $\pm$ 23 b/m.

TABLE 1.   Heart Rate at Exercise Test and
                  Various Daily Life Activities

	Ergometry	Driving	Physical Exertion	Sex	Sleep	At Work	T.V.
$\bar{x}$ H.R.	131.9	106.2	117.1	122.7	77.4	100.6	87.5
$\pm$S.D.	$\pm$20.3	$\pm$23.1	$\pm$21.1	$\pm$23.1	$\pm$18.3	$\pm$21.0	$\pm$21.0

b)   During the 50 minutes calisthenic training, which is a
      part of our rehabilitation program, the mean heart rate
      for the group was 117 $\pm$ 21 b/m (51 patients).

c)   29 patients out of the 75 were recorded during marital
      sexual intercourse, the mean HR was 122 $\pm$23 b/m.

d)   62 patients out of the group were tested during daily
      work, which consisted almost entirely of desk activities
      (managers, accountants, lawyers, etc.). The HR during
      work was 100 $\pm$21 b/m.

e)   47 patients out of the group were tested during leisure
      time which was spent mostly in front of a television set,
      especially during crime films. The mean HR reached
      was 87 $\pm$ 21b/m.

f)   72 patients were recorded during sleep and the mean peak
      HR was 77 $\pm$18 b/m.

3.   Ventricular Ectopic Activity (VEA)

(i)   18.4% of the angina group and 22.2% without angina experienced
       VEA at rest (recorded in a 3 minutes, 12 leads, resting EKG).

(ii)   During exercise, in 21.1% of the patients with A.P. VEA
       was found whereas in 27.7% of patients withou A.P.

(iii) In 67.7% of the whole group VEA was disclosed during
       Holter monitoring. (see table 2).

TABLE 2.   Ventricular Ectopic Activity

	Rest	Exercise	Holter
Patients with A.P.	18.4%	21.1%	
Patients without A.P.	22.2%	27.7%	67.7%

a) In 40 patients recorded during driving, 52.5% developed VEA,
    while in the same patients only 20% had VEA during ergometry.
    27.5% experienced VEA in both situations.

b) In the 29 patients recorded during sex activity, VEA was
    experienced in 34.5% while in stress testing it was experienced
    by 55.1%. in 10.3% VEA was recorded during both situations.

c) In 32 patients recorded during daily work activities, 90.6%
    developed VEA, while only 9.4% had ventricular premature
    contractions during stress testing.

d) 22 patients were recorded during leisure time (TV). 86.3%
    had VEA while watching crime films, only 4.3% of these patients
    had VEA during stress testing. 9.1% had VEA at both situations.

e) In a group of 8 patients who had tachycardias and/or
    tachyarrhythmia, during the majority of daily activities, beta
    blocking compounds such as Propranolol and Oxyprenolol in
    relatively low dosage were administered for several weeks.

Holter recording was repeated during treatment and a significant
decrease in HR and VEA was found. (Because of the small number
of patients involved statistical assessment was not possible).

TABLE 3.   Detection of VEA during Stress and Holter
                    Recording (percent)

Variable Event	N	VEA	VEA During Ergometry	VEA During Event Ergometry
Driving	40	52.5	20.0	27.5
Sex	29	34.5	55.1	10.3
Desk Work	32	90.6	9.4	–
Leisure	22	86.3	4.5	9.1

Statistical Evaluation

The mean pulse rate of 75 patients obtained during Holter
recording was statistically assessed in the following seven
different activities: ergometry, driving, calisthenics, sexual
activity, work, leisure and sleep. (see table 4)

TABLE 4.

	Ergometry	Driving	Phy.Act.	Sex	Sleep	Work	T.V.
N	75	66	51	29	72	62	47
Mean	131.9	106.2	117.1	122.7	77.4	100.6	87.5
S.D.	20.3	23.1	21.4	23.1	18.3	21.0	21.0

In order to examine the differences between the mean of heart rate in the various situations, we used the test of "Analysis of Variance for Single Factor with Repeated Measures on the Same Element". For the purpose of analysis data of 55 out of the 75 patients were used, because only patients where at least 3 situations were recorded: Ergometry (E), Driving (D), and Work (W) were chosen. In testing the significance of differences, all data recorded in the three above mentioned situations were used for analysis. It was found according to the E test (9) that the differences between the mean heart rate in the 3 situations were statistically highly significant (p<0.001). Furthermore, we tested the differences between pairs according to the F test (9).

	F	d.f.	p	
E - D	65.2	108	p	0.001
E - W	95.0	108	p	0.001
W - D	2.81	108	p	0.10

The results indicate that the mean heart rate differences between ergometry and driving, ergometry and work, was highly significant (p<0.001), while the difference between work and driving was of low statistical significance (p<0.10).

STUDY II

Comparison of Asymptomatic and Symptomatic Coronary Patients After Myocardial Infarction.

Material

    This study comprises 93 patients after myocardial infarction who are undergoing a continuous supervised rehabilitation program. The patients were divided into two groups according to symptoms (angina pectoris).

RESULTS

A.   42 patients were asymptomatic with a mean age 52.9 ± 5 years.

    1.   Submaximal Ergometric Test. The submaximal H.R. obtained in 42 asymptomatic patients was 135.4 ± 26.5 b/m. The mean PWC for the group was 88.2 Watt ± 23, 77% of the norm of healthy male individual. The mean target double product was 24.000.

         VEA was present during the exercise test in 14.6% but only 9.7% of the patients had VEA also during one of the daily activity events.

    2.   Heart Rate Holter Recording

        a)   During driving under heavy traffic conditions the mean HR was 90.8 ± 10.2 b/m.

        b)   During physical exertion such as calisthenics, walking, climbing stairs etc. The mean HR was 105.3 ± 22.8 b/m.

        c)   34 out of the 42 patients were recorded during desk work. The mean HR reached was 85.6 ± 24.6 b/m.

        d)   26 out of the 42 patients were recorded during leisure time activity, mostly watching T.V. The mean HR was 82 ± 14.7 b/m.

        e)   During sleeping the mean HR was 56 ± 8.7 b/m.

    3.   Ventricular Ectopic Activity

        (i)   54.0% of the group experienced VEA at rest and in 10.2% VEA was present also at ergometry.

        (ii)   During driving 52.9% had VEA and 11.7% had VEA during driving and ergometry.

        (iii)   21.2% had VEA during physical exertion and 6.7% had VEA during both, physical exertion and ergometry.

TABLE 5.

DETECTION OF V.E.A. DURING STRESS TESTING AND HOLTER
RECORDING, IN SYMPTOMATIC AND ASYMPTOMATIC CORONARY PATIENTS

(Percents)

VARIABLE ACTIVITY	ASYMPTOMATIC AGE 52.9 ± 5.3 N 42 WATT 88.2 ± 23.0				SYMPTOMATIC AGE 55.8 ± 10.1 N 51 WATT 85.0 ± 25.2			
	N	V.E.A.	V.E.A. DURING EVENT AND ERGOMETRY	$\bar{x}$ H.R. ± S.D.	N	V.E.A.	V.E.A. DURING EVENT AND ERGOMETRY	$\bar{x}$ H.R. ± S.D.
REST	25	54.0	10.2	66.7±14.6	28	46.4	3.6	73.7±11.7
DRIVING	34	52.9	11.7	90.8±10.2	43	32.6	9.3	88.3±9.5
PHYSICAL EXERTION	33	21.2	6.7	105.3±22.8	46	17.3	2.2	116.2±18.6
SLEEP	42	33.3	9.5	56.0±8.7	49	28.6	8.2	48.3±8.0
DESK-WORK	34	52.9	8.8	85.6±24.6	42	38.1	4.8	84.6±24.0
LEISURE (T.V. ETC)	26	46.2	7.7	82.0±14.7	26	34.6	11.5	78.5±11.3
ERGOMETRY	41	14.6	9.7	135.4±26.5	49	10.2	10.2	128.6±25.3

(iv)   52.9% experienced VEA while working at their office
       8.8% during both, desk work and ergometry.

(v)   At leisure 46.2% had VEA and 7.7% during leisure
       and ergometry.

(vi)   VEA was connected with sleeping in 33.3% and
       9.5% had VEA during both sleeping and ergometry.

B.   51 patients were symptomatic with mean age 55.8 $\pm$ 10.1 years.

1.   Submaximal Ergometric Test

The submaximal HR obtained in 51 symptomatic patients was
128.6 $\pm$ 25.3 b/min. The mean PWC for the group was 85.0
$\pm$ 25.2, 75% of the norm of healthy male individual. The
mean target double product was 21.000.

VEA was present during the exercise test in 10.2%, and
10.2% of the patients had VEA also during one of the
daily activity events.

2.   Heart Rate Holter Recording

a)   During driving under heavy traffic conditions the
      mean HR was 88.3 $\pm$ 9.5 b/min.

b)   During physical exertion such as calisthenics,
      walking climbing stairs etc. The mean HR was
      116.2 $\pm$ 18.6 b/min.

c)   42 out of the 51 patients were recorded during
      desk work. The mean HR reached was 84.6 $\pm$ 24.0 b/min.

d)   26 out of 51 patients were recorded during leisure
      time activity, mostly watching T.V. The mean HR
      was 78.5 $\pm$ 11.3 b/min.

e)   During sleeping the mean HR was 48.3 $\pm$ 8.0 b/min.

3.   Ventricular Ectopic Activity

(i)   46.4% of the group experienced VEA at rest and in
       3.6% VEA was present also at ergometry.

(ii)   During driving 32.6% had VEA and 9.3% had VEA
       during driving and ergometry.

(iii) 17.3% had VEA during physical exertion and 2.2%
       had VEA during both, physical exertion and ergometry.

   (iv)   38.1% experienced VEA while working at their office
        and 4.8% during both, desk-work and ergometry.

   (v)   At leisure 34.6% had VEA and 11.5% during leisure
        and ergometry.

   (vi)   VEA was connected with sleeping in 28.6% and
        8.2% had VEA during both, sleeping and ergometry.

DISCUSSION

In the present study we have compared incidence and frequency
of VEA during exercise stress testing and 24 hours Holter monitoring.
During stress testing a mean HR of 131 $\pm$ 20 was reached, despite
the fact that mean heart rates of the different daily activities
were significantly lower (p<0.001, VEA appeared more often during
the latter situation. This finding may point to the fact that
gradual, controlled increases in work loads and the performance of
isodynamic exercise do not represent a trigger mechanism for
the appearance of VEA. On the other hand, it must be mentioned
that the 75 patients involved, were participating in a supervised
rehabilitation program which includes systematic physical
training. According to Blackburn et al, (5), progressive
conditioned exercise in previously sedentary men cause a diminition
of the frequency of premature ventricular complexes. Blackburn's
observation may prove important as a beneficial adjunct of the
effect of physical training programs in coronary patients. The
present paper dealing with trained individuals shows, that despite
their enhanced physical work performance VEA occur more often during
their daily life activities. The conclusions of these findings
suggest that physical training as a part of comprehensive
rehabilitation does not protect the patient in patho-physiological
electrical responses to sympathetic stimulation involved in
psychosocial and environmental stresses of daily life. It may be
that training per se will reduce the appearance of VEA during
exercise stress testing, but it probably does not influence the
extent of ventricular dysrhythmias appearing as a result of mental
exertion.

Kosowsky et al. (7) reported that in 27% of their 66 patients
dysrhythmia was disclosed during prolonged monitoring (mostly
14 hours), while in 39% during exercise.

Ryan et al (6) found a higher exposure of VEA during
monitoring, when compared to maximal stress testing.

It is obvious that the appearance of dysrhythmia during
exercise in coronary patients is increased. Dynamic exercise
increases the cardiac output, the stroke volume and linearily the
heart rate and oxygen consumption. A similar hemodynamic response

is obtained during moderate exercise or up to the individual
physiologic adaptability in coronary patients when compared to
healthy individuals. During strenuous exercise however, inadequate
oxygen supply will cause a decrease of myocardial contractility
and function, and therefore may result in electrical instability.

Psychological stresses experienced during normal daily life
activities,often result in a sudden increase in HR which has been
shown to be associated with a large increase in circulating
catecholamines and hyperlipidemia (8).

Kent et al (12) in a study on electrical stability on
acutely ischemic myocardium concluded, that increasing heart rate
within physiologic range by diminishing vagal tone during myocardial
ischemia decreases the electrical stability of the ventrical by
(a) increasing ischemia consequent to the rate induced increase
in myocardial oxygen requirements, and (b) a direct electrophysiologic action of the vagus on the ventricular myocardium. In
the absence of vagal stimulation ventricular fibrillation threshold
was lowered only in one of four dogs, as heart rate was increased
from 50 to 90 beats but decreased 40% as heart rate reached 120
beats, and 74% at 180 beats/min. When vagal stimulation used to
control heart rate ventricular fibrillation threshold was lowered
37% as heart rate was increased from 50 to 60 to 90 beats/min.

Lown et al (11) studied the role of psychologic stress and
autonomic nervous system and the provocation of VEA.   19
patients with advanced grades of VEA were examined by a
psychologic stress which consisted of mental arithemetic reading
from coloured cards and recounting. Autonomic reflex testing
was also studied in 14 of 19 patients. It was concluded that (a)
Objective psychologic test may precipitate ventricular arrhythmia
in susceptible patients, and (b) Evocation of peripheral autonomic
reflexes is an insufficient trigger for enhanced ventricular
ectopic activity.

It is rather difficult to measure objectively mental stress
during daily routine activities.

By means of 24 hours monitoring, one can make only indirect
assessment when sudden appearances of tachycardia and/or
dysrhythmia concur with the patient's protocol indicating stressful
situations. In most of our patients this comparison suggested that
the appearance of tachycardia was often accompanied by VEA. In a
few patients the recorded VEA showed R on T premature contractions,
couples and short runs of VT. To our knowledge the prognostic
significance of VEA, especially those appearing during exercise
and emotional stress, is not yet conclusive. We agree with others
(10) that the neural and psychological inputs together with
various environmental factors may trigger the development of

dysrhythmias and that these mechanisms are unpredictable and uncontrollable. Nevertheless, it is our opinion that one should try to avoid risk of sudden increase in cardiac frequency during daily life activities, as demonstrated in our study. Beta-blocking compounds proved to have a beneficial effect in patients suffering from high frequency induced VEA and tachycardia.

In conclusion: The most important findings of our study indicates that the appearance of VEA was more pronounced during daily life activities when compared to exercise stress testing. Despite a higher target HR during the exercise test, VEA proved to be more frequent at mean heart rates, which were lower than the exercise induced acceleration of heart rate. Another finding was the relatively high appearance of VEA during sleep. In some cases ventricular tachycardia appeared and was probably connected with dreaming. This again would point to the fact that - contrarily to former concepts sleep is a dynamic process connected with arrhythmogenic properties. (14) Finally, we should like to point out that the present study showed a higher incidence of VEA in the asymptomatic group when compared to symptomatic patients, especially during driving, desk work and leisure time activities.

Further follow up may disclose whether or not our findings are of any prognostic importance especially in regard to the effectiveness of an antiarrhythmic therapy.

The fact that only a small percentage of our examinees had VEA both during ergometry and daily life events may be interpreted as a poor correlation between exercise induced VEA on one hand and VEA induced daily routine on the other hand. Naturally it must be taken into consideration that all of our patients (168) were trained individuals and therefore the incidence of VEA during stress testing may have been decreased.

Acknowledgement:

The authors wish to thank Ms. J. Rainitz and A. Lavie for the important technical assistance and Ms. S. Silberwasser for statistical assessment of the results.

References

1. J. J. Kellermann, Rehabilitation of Patients with Coronary Heart Disease. Progress in Cardiovascular Disease, Vol.XVII, No.4 303-327 (1975).
2. J. J. Kellermann, S. Feldman, M. Levi, I. Kariv. Rehabilitation of Coronary Patients. J. Chron. Dis. 20:815-821 (1967).

3. J. J. Kellermann, E. Ben-Ari, M. Chayet, C. Lapidot, Y. Drory and E. Fisman. Cardiocirculatory Response of Different Types of Training in Patients with Angina Pectoris. Cardiology 62:218-231 (1977).

4. J. J. Kellermann, Rehabilitation of Coronary Patients - Experiences. Proceedings of the International Conference on Sports Cardiology, Rome 1978.

5. H. Blackburn, H. L. Taylor, B. Hamrell, W. C. Nicholas, R. D. Thorsen. Premature Ventricular Complexes Induced by Stress Testing. Am. J. Cardiol. 31:441-449 (1973).

6. M. Ryan, B. Lown, H. Horn. Comparison of Ventricular Ectopic Activity During 24 hours Monitoring and Exercise Testing in Patients with Coronary Heart Disease. N.Engl. J. Med. 292:224-229 (1975).

7. B. D. Kosowsky, B. Lown, R. Whiting, T. Cuiney. Occurrence of Ventricular Arrhythmias with Exercise as Compared to Monitoring. Circulation Vol.XLIV, 826-832 (1971).

8. S. H. Taylor. Stress, Hypertension and Beta-Blockade. Modulation of the Circulatory Response to Stress by Beta-Adrenoreceptor Antagonists. IN: "Hypertension - Its Nature and Treatment", Proceedings of an internation symposium Malta, pp.269-282 (1974).

9. B. J. Winter. "Statistical Principles in Experimental Design" McGraw Hill Book Comp. Inc. (1962).

10. B. Lown, M. Tykociniski, A. Garfein et al. Sleep and Ventricular Premature Beats. Circulation 48:691-701 (1973).

11. B. Lown, R. A. DeSilva and R. Lenson. Roles of psychologic stress and automatic system changes in provocation of ventricular premature complexes. The American Journal of Cardiology 41:979-985 (1978).

12. K. M. Kent, E. R. Smith, B. R. Redwood and S. E. Epstein. Electrical stability of acutely ischemic myocardium. Circulation XLVII: 291-297 (1973).

13. J. J. Kellerman, Modulated sympathetic stimulation as a desirable feature within the framework of comprehensive rehabilitation in patients with coronary heart disease. In: "Modulation of sympathetic tone in the treatment of cardio-vascular diseases", F. Gross ed., Proc. Inter. Symp. Manila (1978); Huber Verlag, Basel.

14. G. A. Winkle, D. C. Derrington and J. S. Schroeder. Characteristics of Ventricular tachycardia in ambulatory patients. The American Journal of Cardiology, 39:487-492 (1977).

CLINICAL SIGNIFICANCE OF CARDIAC ARRHYTHMIAS DETECTED DURING EXERCISE

Ezra A. Amsterdam, Anthony D. DeMaria, Lawrence J. Laslett, and Dean T. Mason

Section of Cardiovascular Medicine
Departments of Medicine and Physiology
University of California
School of Medicine and Sacramento Medical Center
Davis and Sacramento, California

Disturbances of cardiac rhythm are commonly observed during exercise testing and may provide information of diagnostic, prognostic and therapeutic importance (1-7). Data demonstrating an association between ventricular ectopy and increased risk of cardiac disease and sudden death have stimulated interest in the clinical significance of exercise-induced ventricular arrhythmias. This chapter will review the electrophysiologic response of the cardio-circulatory system to exercise and current knowledge of the significance of exercise-induced arrhythmias in the identification and prognosis of cardiac disease.

EFFECTS OF EXERCISE ON CARDIAC RHYTHM

Exercise is capable of inducing a number of alterations in the electrical activity of the myocardium, the net result of which may be either enhancement or inhibition of ectopic rhythms and abnormal conduction. Derangement of cardiac electrophysiology as a response of exercise is unpredictable in an individual subject, and cardiac rhythm and conduction may vary as a function of the level of exertion or stress. Figure 1 illustrates physiologic alterations accompanying exercise and their possible sequelae.

Pathophysiology of Exercise-Induced Arrythmias

The stress of exertion frequently results in the appearance of arrhythmias not present in the resting state. The production of such arrhythmias by exercise has been attributed to heightened

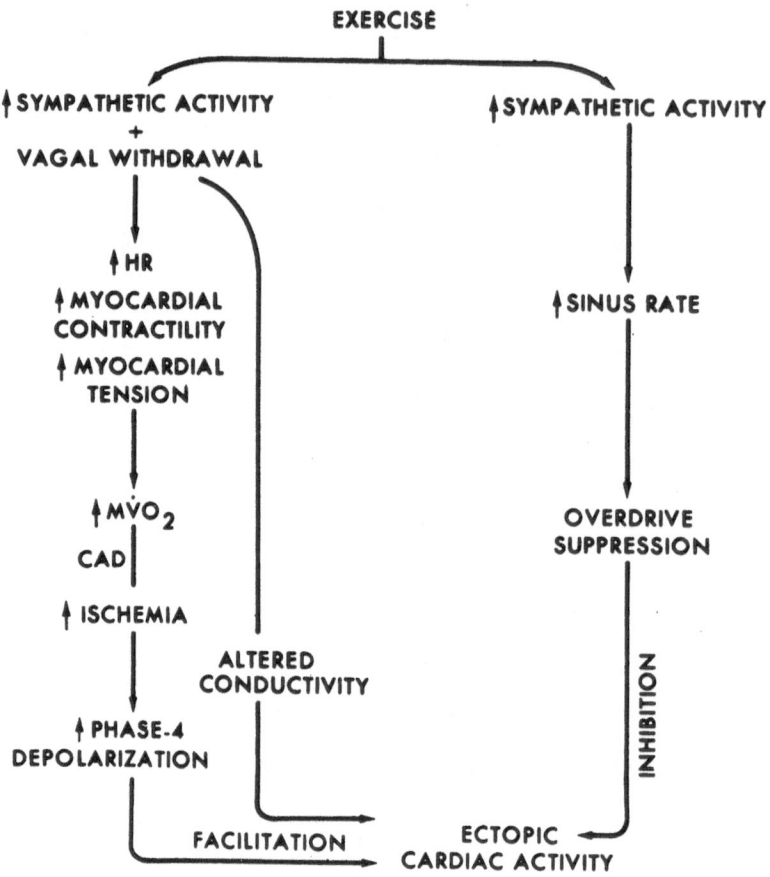

Figure 1.

sympathetic tone, increased myocardial oxygen demand or a
combination of these factors. Augmented sympathetic drive to the
myocardium may provoke ectopic Purkinje pacemaker activity by
accelerating the rate of phase-4 depolarization at this site,
enhancing its spontaneous discharge and thereby increasing
automaticity (8,9). Increased myocardial oxygen demand, when
not matched by oxygen supply, results in local tissue hypoxia.
Myocardial hypoxia produces temporal dispersion of depolarization
and repolarization as well as alterations in conduction velocity
and thereby provides a substrate for the appearance of arrhythmias
related to both automaticity and reentry (10). Thus, myocardial
ischemia may act as the stimulus for the appearance of abnormalities
of rhythm and conduction during stress testing. Myocardial
fibrosis or dilatation as occurs in coronary, valvular, primary

myocardial or inflammatory cardiac lesions may also provide a
pathologic basis for enhanced automaticity and reentry mechanisms
which provoke arrhythmias during stress testing.

Myocardial ischemia is a common response to exercise stress
in the presence of coronary artery disease. Myocardial oxygen
consumption ($M\dot{V}O_2$) is determined by heart rate, contractility and
intramyocardial tension (11). The effect of exercise upon these
factors augments $M\dot{V}O_2$ and thus may result in myocardial ischemia
if oxygen demand exceeds supply. This disparity is usually a
consequence of the restricted flow reserve of the coronary
circulation in coronary atherosclerotic disease. Such an
imbalance may be related not only to elevated levels of exercise
stress, but also to events in the immediate postexercise period.
At this time, peripheral arteriolar dilatation induced by exercise,
and reduced cardiac output resulting from diminished venous return
secondary to the abrupt cessation of muscular activity, may
combine to produce a reduction in blood pressure and decreased
coronary perfusion while the heart rate is still increased. Thus,
arrhythmias may occur during exercise in normal or diseased hearts
due to the interaction between the myocardium and the neurohumoral
concomitants of exertional stress. The type of arrhythmia and the
level of exercise by which it is provoked aid in determining its
clinical significance. These factors will be considered later in
this chapter.

Reduction of Arrhythmias by Exercise: Although the pre-
cipitation of arrythmias by exercise is widely recognized,
abolition during exercise of ectopic cardiac activity present at
rest is a less appreciated phenomenon. The ability of exercise
to abolish arrhythmias present in the resting state has generally
been attributed to two mechanisms, both of which are related to
the sinus tachycardia resulting from vagal withdrawal and increased
sympathetic stimulation accompanying exercise. Thus, sinus
tachycardia may inhibit an ectopic focus before its intrinsic
discharge reaches threshold potential, an example of overdrive
suppression. In addition, there is evidence that rapid stimulation
may result in decreased automaticity of Purkinje tissue and thus
sinus tachycardia may inhibit automaticity of an ectopic
focus (12).

EXERCISE-INDUCED ALTERATIONS OF RHYTHM AND CONDUCTION

Supraventricular Arrhythmias: A wide variety of supraventricular arrhythmias may be noted in the process of stress
testing. Wandering or ectopic atrial pacemakers and sinus
arrhythmias are particularly common after exercise (5).
However, although 3 to 5 beat episodes of paroxysmal atrial and
junctional tachyarrhythmias occurred frequently during exertion in
3,000 patients studied by Gooch, sustained bouts lasting more than

15 seconds occurred in only 5 patients (5). Several investigators
(2-5) have noted that atrial fibrillation and flutter are only
rarely induced by exertion and, when they do occur, revert spontaneously. Indeed, observation of the response of ventricular rate to various levels of activity has provided an excellent method of assessing
adequacy of digitalization in patients with atrial fibrillation (13).
This response could not be predicted from the resting heart rate. Finally rare episodes of sinoatrial block and sinus arrest have been noted
during stress testing, usually after termination of exercise (5).

Conduction Defects: Alterations of cardiac conduction
involving both the atrioventricular (AV) node and bundle branches
may occur during the course of exercise testing. AV conduction is
accelerated during exertion under normal circumstances (14) and
absence of such shortening has been regarded as an abnormal
response indicative of AV junctional block. In addition, the
appearance of frank first degree heart block or its progression to
more advanced block has also been noted in association with
exercise (2-5). Conversely, preexisting block of the AV node has
been noted to decrease in this setting, a phenomenon that may be
related to enhanced conduction velocity due to increased sympathetic
stimulation.

Abnormalities of ventricular conduction consisting of intra-
ventricular conduction defects and bundle branch block involving
either the left or right bundle branch were observed in 8 of 733
patients undergoing stress testing (5). Seven of these eight
patients had clinical evidence of heart disease. Sandberg (2)
reported a small group of patients who manifested bundle branch
block during exertion and in whom the appearance of the defect with
mild effort was associated with clinical evidence of cardiac disease.
In both of the latter studies the abnormalities of conduction were
usually preceded by evidence of incomplete block in the resting
electrocardiogram, and they appeared during exercise and disappeared
after termination of the stress.

Ventricular Arrhythmias: Ectopic beats and tachyarrhythmias
of ventricular origin have been frequently described during exercise
testing (15-20). Thus, in several studies (15-18), ventricular arrhythmias with exertion were noted in from 20% to 49% of patients.
Ectopic ventricular beats were observed most commonly in the postexercise period in all but one study (17) and frequently occurred late in
the recovery period. Thus, two thirds of cessation of exercise and
the single death reported in a large group of patients with coronary
disease occurred suddenly 4 minutes after completion of the exercise
test (15). Salvos of ventricular tachycardia were preceded by single
ectopic beats in the vast majority of cases. Premature ventricular
contractions occurred with increased frequency with advancing age(16)
and higher levels of effort (16,17).

DIAGNOSTIC IMPLICATIONS OF EXERCISE-INDUCED VENTRICULAR ARRHYTHMIAS

Considerable interest has been stimulated in the diagnostic
and prognostic significance of ventricular arrhythmias occurring
during graded bicycle or treadmill exercise testing. Although the
significance of these rhythm disturbances has not been firmly
established, certain patterns seem evident on the basis of the
information currently available.

Debate continues on the significance of exercise-induced
ventricular extrasystoles as indicators of the presence of organic
heart disease. Several early investigations (21-24) demonstrated
the occurrence of ventricular arrhythmias in apparently normal
persons and failed to find a correlation between ventricular
ectopic beats elicited during effort and clinical evidence of
cardiac disease. Sandberg(2) found that the subset of patients
who demonstrated ventricular arrhythmias after light effort also
manifested clinical heart disease, and Gooch and McConnell (1)
related bursts of ventricular tachycardia to the presence of
cardiac abnormalities. These conclusions were supported by
McHentry and associated (16) who, while observing ventricular
ectopy in more than one-third of apparently normal subjects, noted
an even greater frequency of ventricular arrhythmias in patients
with clinically evident or suspected cardiac disease. In the patients
manifesting these abnormalities, ventricular ectopic beats were
provoked by lighter exertion and at lower heart rates and had a
greater tendency to be frequent, multifocal or repetitive.
In all these studies the criteria for heart disease were based upon
clinical evidence; thus, subclinical cardiac abnormalities may well
have been present and undetected in the "normal" group. A
unique criterion suggesting whether or not exercise-induced
premature ventricular beats are related to coronary artery disease
was recently reported by Mardelli et al (25) in a study of 73
patients, all of whom underwent coronary angiography. In all 10
patients without coronary disease the extrasystoles had an axis of
-15° to $+110^{\circ}$. By contrast, a superior axis of -30° to -120° was
present in 76% of the 63 patients with coronary disease.

The diagnostic significance of exercise-induced ventricular
extrasystoles in an asymptomatic polulation has been clarified by
the study of Froelicher et al in which 1390 apparently healthy men
were followed for a mean period of 6.3 years and end-points of
angina, myocardial infarction and sudden death (8) were correlated
with ventricular arrhythmias occurring during exercise (26).
Ventricular extrasystoles developing during exercise were classified
as "ominous" if frequent ($\geq$20% of any series of 50 beats),
occuring in couplets with other ectopy that arose during exercise
or occurring in salvos of three or more. "Ominous" ventricular
extrasystoles developed in 2.1% of subjects and their occurrence
was directly related to age: age 20-29 years - 0.8% had "ominous"

ventricular extrasystoles; 30-39 years - 1.0%; 40-53 years - 3.5%.
Although subjects with "ominous" arrhythmias had a risk of
developing coronary heart disease during the 6.3 year post-test
period that was 3.4 times (risk ratio) that of subjects without
these arrhythmias, the prognostic value of these arrhythmias was
limited by a low sensitivity (6.7%) and predictive value (10%);
that is, only 6.7% of those developing a coronary heart disease
end-point had "ominous" arrhythmias and only 10% of individuals
with the "ominous" arrhythmias developed a disease end-point.

     Zaret et al (27) evaluated exercise-induced ventricular
irritability in a group of patients undergoing coronary arteriography and found coronary atherosclerosis in 72%. Multiple
vessel coronary disease was significantly more common than in
matched patients without arrhythmias. Goldschlager et al (15)
compared a group of patients with ventricular arrhythmias elicited
by exertion with patients without such disturbances who had under-
gone cardiac catheterization and coronary arteriography. These
investigatiors found significant coronary stenosis in 89% of
exercise-precipitated ventricular extrasystoles. In addition,
they observed a significantly greater prevalence of double and
triple vessel coronary artery disease and abnormal left ventricular
wall motion in this group than in patients with coronary heart
disease without arrhythmias. Provoked arrhythmias occurred more
frequently during the recovery period in this study. A striking
finding was the disappearance of ectopic beats during exercise
stress in a high percentage of patients with significant coronary
disease. Morris and McHenry (6) have provided an important
demonstration of the relationship between, on the one hand, the
presence and severity of coronary disease and, on the other, the
type of arrhythmia and the level of exercise at which it is
provoked. They found that at heart rates less than 70% of
predicted maximum, only 7% of 285 normal individuals had ventricular
arrhythmias whereas ventricular ectopy occurred in 27% of the
197 patients with coronary disease (P<0.001). The coronary group
manifested a significantly higher frequency of multifocal
ventricular extrasystoles, runs of ventricular tachycardia and
frequent (>10/min) ventricular extrasystoles. Further, within the
coronary disease group, the occurrence of exercise-induced
ventricular arrhythmias was significantly greater in patients with
multi-vessel coronary involvement and/or left ventricular wall
motion abnormalities.

     The relationship between exercise and ventricular arrhythmias
in patients with coronary heart disease was also investigated by
Helfant et al(20). They observed that ventricular extrasystoles
appeared or were increased in frequency with exercise in 22 of 38
patients with coronary atherosclerosis; the vast majority of these
patients manifested multivessel coronary disease and ventricular
asynergy. It was noteworthy that 20 or the 22 patients in this

study who exhibited exercise-related arrhythmias also manifested evidence of myocardial ischemia by virtue of the development of 2 mm or greater ST-segment depression. However, other investigators have not observed a similar relationship between exercise-induced arrhythmias and ST-segment depression.

It is important to appreciate that ventricular arrhythmias associated with exertion are a non-specific finding and that the presence of "serious" rhythm disturbances at low levels of exertion, while suggestive of organic heart disease, does not necessarily indicate coronary involvement. Thus, in the presence of normal coronary arteries, valvular heart disease associated with impairment of cardiac function may result in exercise-induced rhythm disturbances on the basis of the mechanisms previously enumerated.

Although ventricular arrhythmias occur in the absence of organic heart disease, certain conclusions appear justified from the findings cited:

1.   Ventricular arrhythmias provoked by exertion occur significantly more frequently in patients who have cardiac disease than in normal subjects;

2.   Ventricular ectopic beats that occur at exercise heart rates of $\leq 70\%$ of predicted maximum rate, or demonstrate high frequency, multifocal patterns or repetitive firing are particularly suggestive of cardiac disease;

3.   Patients with coronary atherosclerosis who have ventricular rhythm disorders induced by stress testing have a greater frequency of multiple vessel coronary disease and abnormalities of ventricular wall motion;

4.   The termination of ventricular ectopy during exertion does not indicate the absence of flow-limiting coronary atherosclerosis;

5.   Exercise-induced ventricular arrhythmias are a non-specific finding and can occur in any type of cardiac disease as well as in normals.

PROGNOSTIC SIGNIFICANCE OF VENTRICULAR ARRHYTHMIAS OCCURING DURING EXERCISE

Premature ventricular contractions manifested in a resting electrocardiogram (28,29) or during activity (30) have been associated with an increased incidence of coronary atherosclerosis, subsequent mortality and sudden death. The risk is especially prominent in patients with known cardiovascular abnormalities (31). However, the resting electrocardiogram has a substantially lower

yield than exercise electrocardiography in the detection of
ectopic ventricular rhythms (18). It would seem reasonable
that ectopic ventricular beats provoked by exertion might carry
serious prognostic implications and thus be of potential
importance in indicating risk of sudden death.

In contrast to the previously noted low prognostic
sensitivity of ventricular ectopy associated with exercise in
asymptomatic men (26), Morris and McHenry (6) have reported an
important relationship between exercise-induced ventricular
arrhythmias and subsequent sudden death in coronary patients. Of
ten sudden deaths in 260 patients during a mean observation period
of 18 months, eight occurred in the group of 50 patients who
manifested "complex" ventricular arrhythmias at exercise heart
rates of ≤ 130/min. The 16% incidence of sudden death in the latter
subgroup was significantly greater ($P < 0.001$) than that in the
subgroups with absence of or simple ventricular arrhythmias during
exercise. Further longterm data are required to more fully
evaluate the prognostic significance of exercise-induced
arrhythmias in patients with coronary artery disease. However,
exercise-elicited ventricular extrasystoles have already been
correlated with the coronary risk factors of hypertension and
glucose intolerance as well as with ischemic electrocardiographic
abnormalities and enlargement of the cardiac silhouette on
roentgenographic study (3). Indeed, in this study population,
sudden death occurred in two patients with exertional ventricular
irritability. That such potential disasters may be amenable to
therapy is suggested by Bryson et al (4), who reported in three
patients, exertional ventricular tachycardia and fibrillation which
prompted coronary arteriography revealing significant coronary
atherosclerosis. Subsequently these exercise-provoked arrhythmias
were abolished by coronary artery bypass surgery.

SUMMARY

Although a wide spectrum of cardiac rhythm disturbances occur
with exercise, ventricular arrhythmias are of greatest frequency
and importance. Exertion may induce arrhythmias as a result of
neurohumoral stimulation and myocardial factors which result in
abnormalities of automaticity and reentry phenomena. Exercise
may abolish arrhythmias present in the resting state by overdrive
suppression and inhibition related to sinus tachycardia.
Ventricular premature beats occur commonly in apparently healthy
individuals as well as in patients with cardiac disease but
ventricular ectopy that is frequent, multifocal or repetitive and
provoked by low exercise levels is strongly suggestive of cardiac
disease. Most studies have related the latter factors to
coronary disease but exercise-induced ventricular arrhythmias are
a non-specific finding and may be associated with any type of
significant cardiac pathology. Exertional ventricular irritability

occurs with increased frequency in patients with multi-vessel coronary disease and abnormalities of left ventricular wall motion. Abolition of resting ventricular ectopy by exercise does not exclude the presence of cardiac disease.

REFERENCES

1. A. S. Gooch, D. McConnel, Analysis of transient arrhythmias and conduction disturbances occurring during submaximal treadmill exercise testing. Prog Cardiovasc Dis, 13:293-307(1970).
2. L. Sandberg, The significance of ventricular premature beats or runs of ventricular tachycardia developing during exercise tests, Acta. Med. Scand., 169:1-117 (1961).
3. J. A. Vedin, C. E. Wilhelmsson, et al, Relations of resting and exercise-induced ectopic beats to other ischemic manifestations and to coronary risk factors. Men born in 1913, Amer. J. Cardiol., 30:25-31 (1972).
4. A. L. Bryson, A. F. Oarisi, E. Schecter, et al, Life threatening arrhythmias induced by exercise cessation after coronary bypass surgery, Amer. J. Cardiol., 30:25-31 (1972).
5. A. S. Gooch, Exercise testing for detecting changes in cardiac rhythm and conduction. Amer. J. Cardiol. 30:741-746 (1972).
6. S. N. Morris, P. L. McHenry, Cardiac Arrhythmias during Exercise Testing and Exercise Conditioning, in N. K. Wenger (ed), Exercise and the Heart, p. 57-68 (1978), F. A. Davis, Philadelphia.
7. N. Goldschlager, K. Cohn, A. Goldschlager, Exercise-related ventricular arrhythmias. Mod. Con. Cardiov. Dis., 48:67 (1979).
8. M. Vassalle, M. J. Levine, J. H. Stuckey, Sympathetic control of ventricular automaticity,: the effects of stellate ganglion stimulation. Circ. Res., 23:249-258 (1968).
9. M. Vassalle, J. H. Stuckey, M. J. Levine, Sympathetic control of ventricular automaticity: role of the adrenal medulla, Amer. J. Physiol., 217:930-937 (1969).
10. M. R. Rosen, B. F. Hoffman, Mechanisms of action of antiarrhythmic drugs. Circ. Res., 32:1-8 (1973).
11. E. H. Sonnenblick, C. L. Skelton, Oxygen consumption of the heart: physiologic principles and clinical implications, Mod. Concepts Cardiovasc. Dis., 40:9-16 (1971).
12. J. Alanis, D. Benitez, The decrease in the automatism of the Purkinje pacemaker fibers provoked by high frequencies of stimulation, Jap. J. Physiol., 17:556-571 (1967).
13. A. S. Gooch, G. Natarajan, J. Goldberg, Influence of exercise on arrhythmias induced by digitalis-diuretic therapy in patients with atrial fibrillation, Amer. J. Cardiol., 33:230: 237 (1974).

14. J. W. Lister, E. Stein, B. D. Kosowsky, et al, Atrioventricular conduction in man. Effect of rate, exercise isoproterenol and atropine on the P-R interval, Amer. J. Cardiol., 16:516-523 (1966).

15 N. Goldschlager, D. Cake, K. Cohn, Exercise-induced ventricular arrhythmias in patients with coronary artery disease. Their relation to angiographic findings, Amer. J. Cardiol., 31:434-440 (1973).

16. P. L. McHenry, G. Fisch, J. W. Jordan, et al, Cardiac arrhythmias observed during maximal exercise testing in clinically normal men, Amer. J. Cardiol., 29:331-336 (1972).

17. H. Blackburn, H. L. Taylor, H. Burtram, et al, Premature ventricular complexes induced by stress testing. Their frequency and response to physical conditioning, Amer. J. Cardiol., 31:441-449 (1973).

18. B. D. Kosowsky, B. Lown, R. Whiting, et al, The occurrence of ventricular arrhythmias with exercise as compared to monitoring, Circulation 44:826-832 (1971).

19. M. Ryan, B. Lown, H. Horn, Comparison of ventricular ectopic activity during 24-hour monitoring and exercise testing in patients with coronary heart disease, New Eng. J. Med., 292:224-229 (1975).

20. R. Helfant, R. Pine, V. Kadbe, V. Banka, Exercise-related ventricular premature complexes in coronary heart disease, Ann. Intern. Med., 80:589-592 (1974).

21. L. E. Lamb, H. B. Burcheil, Premature ventricular contractions and exercise, Proc. Staff Meet. Mayo Clin., 27:383-389 (1952).

22. A. M. Master, I. Rosenfelt, Two-step exercise test: current status after twenty-five years, Mod. Concepts Cardiovasc. Dis., 36:19-24 (1967).

23. T. W. Mattingly, The postexercise electrocardiogram, Amer. J. Cardiol., 9:395-409 (1962).

24. L. T. Sheffield, J. H. Holt, T. J. Reeves, Exercise graded by heart rate in electrocardiographic testing for angina pectoris, Circulation 32:622-629 (1965).

25. T. J. Mardell, J. Morganroth, L. S. Dreifus, Superior QRS axis of ventricular premature complexes: an additional criterion to enhance the sensitivity of exercise stress testing, Amer. J. Cardiol., 45:236 (1980).

26. V. F. Froelicher, M. Thomas, C. Pillow, et al., An epidemiological study of asymptomatic men screened with exercise testing for latent coronary heart disease, Am. J. Cardiol., 34:770 (1974).

27. B. L. Zaret, C. R. Conti Jr., Exercise-induced ventricular irritability: hemodynamic and angiographic correlation (abstract), Amer. J. Cardiol., 29:298 (1972).

28. B. M. Chiang, L. V. Perlman, L. D. Ostrander Jr., et al, Relation of premature systoles to coronary heart disease and sudden death in the Tecumseh epidemiologic study, Ann. Intern. Med., 70:1159-1166 (1969).

29. H. Blackburn, H. L. Taylor, A. Keyes, The electrocardiogram
     in prediction of five-year coronary heart disease incidence
     among men aged forty through fifty-nine. Circulation 41
     (suppl I):154-161 (1970).
30. L. E. Hinkle Jr., S. T. Carver, M. Stevens, The frequency of
     asympomatic disturbances of cardiac rhythm and conduction in
     middle-aged men, Amer. J. Cardiol., 24:629-650 (1969).
31. M. Rodstein, L. Wollock, R. Guber, Mortality study of the
     significance of extrasystoles in an insured population,
     Circulation 44:617-625 (1971).

FUNCTIONAL EVALUATION OF PATIENTS WITH IMPLANTED PACEMAKERS

A. Raineri, G. Mercurio, A.M. Milito, and P. Assennato

Cattedra di Fisiopatologia Cardiovascolare
Università di Palermo
Italy

Because of the knowledge that his life is dependent on the pacemaker and due to the uncertainty of some clinical results, the paced patient needs a guide to return to society.

Many studies have attempted to show the ideal heart rate during ventricular pacing in the presence of complete AV heart block. However, most authors agree that rates between 60 and 80 beats per minute appear most ideal (1-6). But during the physical activity the functional condition of the cardiovascular system needs an increased heart rate that the normal pacemaker can't give. It is for this reason that the implanted patient has a different hemodynamic behaviour, and it is necessary to know the guiding criteria in the programme of an ergometric test, and to establish the usefulness of the findings in order to evaluate the patient's physical capacity.

For these reasons we decided to study some of our pacemaker implanted patients.

MATERIALS AND METHODS

28 patients (6 females and 22 males), aged between 33 and 64 (average 52±11SD) have been chosed from 276 pacemaker implanted patients (implanted and followed in our Institute) for the evaluation of their physical capacity.

This chosing was determined by keeping in mind the following factors: patients in a working age, with good cardiac performance, with normal pressure, capable of doing the exercise on the cycle ergometer, at least one year after implantation.

The necessity of the pacemaker was determined by a complete AV block in 26 cases and sick sinus syndrome in 2 cases. A demand type pacemaker with a transvenous electrode and a rate of 72 had been implanted in all cases.

The functional evaluation of the physical capacity had been made with discontinuous cycle ergometer test with 25 watt increasing work load lasting 5 minutes with intermittent rest periods of 5 minutes.

The minute ventilation ($\dot{V}E$), the oxygen consumption* ($\dot{V}O_2$ litres/min), the ECG and the blood pressure were recorded at rest, at the 5th minute of every work load, and at the 5th minute of recovery. The spiroergometer test was interrupted if any of the following occurred:

a)   if $\dot{V}O_2$ did not increase from work load to work load

b)   muscular fatigue

c)   all the remaining criteria that we know for the interruption of the test, except the heart rate.

In 20 patients we recorded simultaneously the thoracic electrical impedance in order to value a possible heart failure. This method infact allows a quantitative evaluation of thoracic fluid volume (7).

15 normal subjects similar in age, sex, occupation had been selected as a control group.

The results have been statistically evaluated. The analysis of variance had been made to assess the behaviour of $\dot{V}O_2$, watts and O_2P among the pacemaker implanted patients groups. The Student's "t" test has been utilized to compare the data in each group of pacemaker implanted patients in respect to control group. The linear regression has been utilized to study the relationship among $\dot{V}O_2$, $\dot{V}E$ and O_2P.

RESULTS

As shown on Table I, 18 patients had at rest pacemaker rhythm. The remaining 10 patients had spontaneous (i.e. junctional or idioventricular rhythm) or sinus rhythm which alternated with the pacemaker.

---

*Biotec Oxitest (Bologna, Italy), open circuit analyser.

TABLE I

Rhythm, heart rate, blood pressure at rest and after exercise in implanted pacemaker patients and control.

RHYTHM	REST			EXERCISE		
	nº	HR beats/min	BP mmHg	nº	HR ±SD beats/min	BP mmHg
PACED	18	72	$\frac{122}{80}$	5	72	$\frac{176}{82}$
SPONTANEOUS	–	–	$\frac{133}{82}$	9	103 ± 14	$\frac{183}{86}$
PACED, SPONTANEOUS OR SINUS	10	80	–	–	–	–
SINUS	–	–	$\frac{128}{85}$	14	124 ± 17	$\frac{180}{88}$
CONTROL	15	78	$\frac{130}{85}$	15	153 ± 15	$\frac{185}{90}$

During the exercise 5 patients remained paced at the proper rate of the pacemaker, i.e. 72 beats/min. In this group the blood pressure at rest was 122/80 mmHg and during the exercise 176/82 mmHg.

The heart rate increased in 9 patients as a result of a spontaneous rhythm starting, which either refers to junctional or idioventricular rhythm. In these cases heart rate was 103±14SD beats/min. Blood pressure at rest was 133/82 mmHg and after exercise 183/86 mmHg.

In the remaining 14 patients sinus rhythm was restored with a rate of 124±17 SD beats/min. The blood pressure was 128/85 at rest and 180/88 mmHg after the exercise. In the control group the heart rate at rest was 78 and after the exercise 153±15 SD beats/min. The blood pressure at rest was 130/85 mmHg and 185/90 mmHg after exercise.

The work load reached (fig. 1) was as follows:

The sinus and spontaneous rhythm patients achieved a work load of 100±17 watts; the paced rhythm patients achieved a work load of 90±13.6 watt; the control group achieved a work load of 108±27 SD watt.

There wasn't any statistical significance in the comparison.

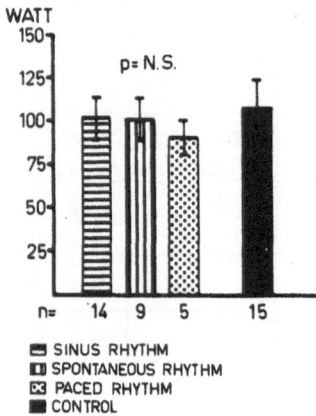

Fig. 1. Mean work load in pacemaker implanted patients and
         control.

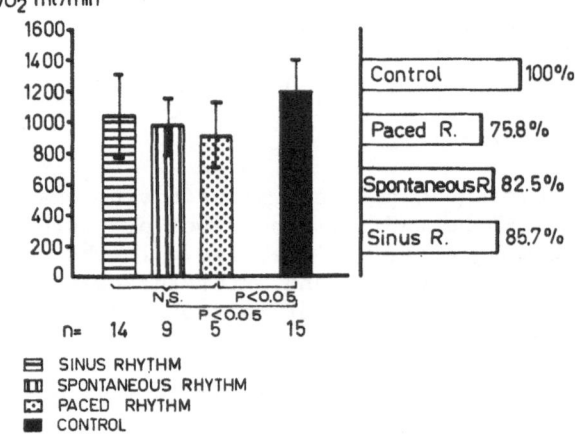

Fig. 2. Mean $\dot{V}O_2$ max. and percent. in pacemaker implanted
         patients and control.

The oxygen consumption (fig. 2) was 1029 ± 289 ml/min in the sinus patients; 990 ± 198 ml/min in the spontaneous rhythm patients; 910 ± 229 SD ml/min in the paced rhythm patients. The oxygen consumption was 1200 ± 226 SD ml/min in the control group.

The group of patients with paced rhythm during exercise had lower aerobic capacity (75.8%) compared with the control group and the other two groups.

The spontaneous rhythm patients had an aerobic capacity of 82.5% compared to the control. The sinus rhythm patients had an aerobic capacity of 85.7%. There isn't any statistical difference among pacemaker implanted patients groups. A statistical significance exists in confronting paced rhythm patients, spontaneous rhythm patients and control.

Fig 3 compares the average values of oxygen consumption at different levels of effort and shows the corresponding heart rates in each group. The sinus rhythm patients performed a work load and oxygen consumption similar to control. The spontaneous rhythm patients, although performing the same work load had a lower aerobic capacity than sinus rhythm patients. The paced rhythm patients had the lowest physical capacity. Heart rate was 72 beats per min. in this group, 103 ± 14 SD beats/min in spontaneous rhythm, 124 ± 17.9 SD in sinus rhythm patients and 153 ± 15 SD in control.

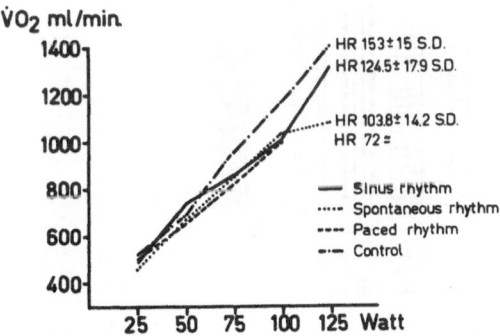

Fig. 3.   Mean $\dot{V}O_2$ at increased work load and heart rate achieved.

These rates correspond to the different oxygen consumptions and work loads.

The mean oxygen pulse (O_2P) in pacemaker implanted patients and in control group (Fig. 4) have shown the following. The paced rhythm patients had a O_2P of 12.21 ± 3 SD; the spontaneous rhythm patients 9.9 ± 2.9 SD; sinus rhythm patients 8.34 ± 2.1 SD; control group 7.8 ± 1.5 SD. A significant difference exists in comparing the three groups of pacemaker implanted patients ($p < 0.05$). There is a remarkable difference ($p < 0.001$) between paced rhythm patients and the control group.

There is no significant difference between sinus rhythm group and control, while there is a significant difference between spontaneous rhythm and control ($p < 0.05$).

The relationship between oxygen consumption and oxygen pulse (fig. 5) is linear and is the same for all groups examined: $r = 0.79$ in paced rhythm; $r = 0.85$ in spontaneous rhythm; $r = 0.84$ in sinus; $r = 0.75$ in control.

In the control group the higher oxygen consumption corresponds to lower oxygen pulse.

This characteristic has a tendency to invert if one observes our groups with sinus rhythm, spontaneous rhythm or paced rhythm.

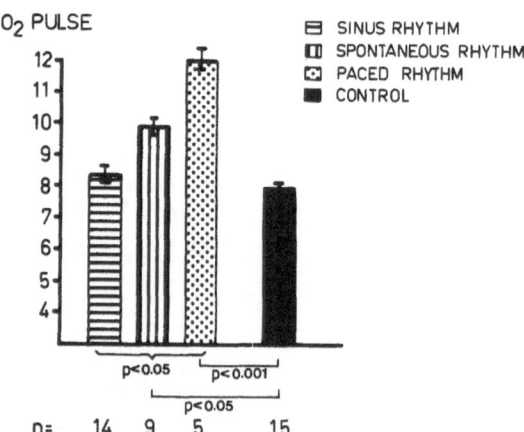

Fig. 4. Mean max O_2 pulse in pacemaker implanted patients and control.

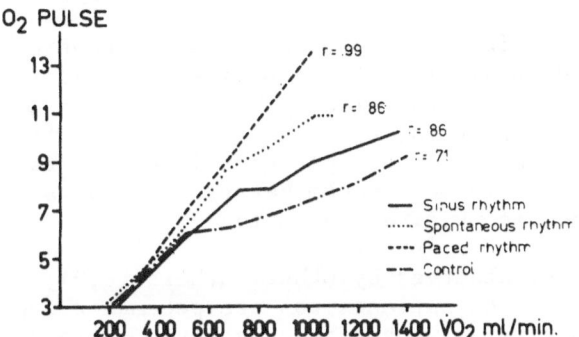

Fig. 5.   Relationship between O_2 pulse and $\dot{V}O_2$ mean values.

In our research we have taken into consideration the
relationship between ventilation and oxygen consumption
(fig. 6). The linear progression is shown by the high value
of r, which is 0.98 on pacemaker implanted patients; 0.99 in
the control group.

The paced rhythm patients show a line with higher slope in
respect to all the other groups; they need more ventilation for
the same oxygen consumption.

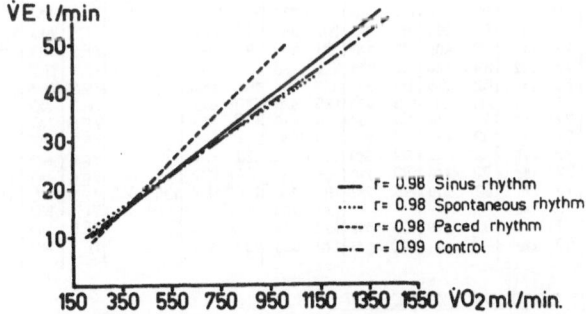

Fig. 6.   Relationship between $\dot{V}E$ and $\dot{V}O_2$ regression lines.

The thoracic electrical impedance did not change after the

Discussion

The pacemaker implanted patients that we have examined can do work loads similar to those of the control group. If we keep in mind that the blood pressure changes during the effort as a normal pattern, and that the clinical findings and the impedance values put these patients in normal range, we can be certain that to be a pacemaker carrier doesn't always mean to be handicapped in physical capacity.

Our findings, observed by other authors (8,9), allows us to distinguish a group of patients who are pacemaker dependents, a group of patients who have spontaneous rhythm with a rate higher than the pacemaker rate, and a group of patients who restore to sinus rhythm. The latter happened in 50% of cases.

The sympathetic acitivity induced by the effort is clearly responsible for these effects. We know for example that the atrial rhythm changes under these conditions in patients with a complete AV block (10,11).

This behaviour shows that in general the heart in paced patients can respond in the same way as normal. But we have noticed that, besides the paced rhythm patients, the changes in heart rate are not completely physiological (Table II).

TABLE II

Work loads, VO_2 and heart rate in 14 patients with restored sinus rhythm. Reasons for discontinuing the test.

AGE years	SEX	REST HR $\dot{V}O_2$		25 W HR $\dot{V}O_2$		50 W HR $\dot{V}O_2$		75 W HR $\dot{V}O_2$		100 W HR $\dot{V}O_2$		125 W HR $\dot{V}O_2$		REASONS FOR DISCONTINUING THE TEST			
														a	b	c	d
55	M	70	214	90	550	100	785	100	830	115	840			YES	NO	YES	YES
55	M	72	182	92	500	92	700	110	980	110	950			YES	NO	YES	YES
64	M	72	246	72	600	72	770	90	900	90	990			YES	NO	YES	?
50	M	76	232	83	580	92	920	105	1160	—	—	150	1500	YES	YES	NO	?
58	M	72	217	82	365	99	800	99	—	165	1200			YES	YES	YES	?
48	M	76	212	100	540	115	730	125	930	130	900			YES	NO	NO	YES
61	M	72	168	72	315	80	650	88	800	110	900			YES	NO	NO	?
64	M	76	330	92	630	110	940	130	1030	—	—			YES	YES	NO	YES
56	M	72	236	—	—	90	690	—	—	120	1170	130	1300	YES	NO	NO	NO
35	M	72	183	72	450	80	710	—	—	94	1300	120	1600	YES	NO	NO	NO
52	M	70	175	83	570	98	785	110	940	125	1140	135	1200	YES	NO	NO	YES
43	F	70	220	—	—	—	—	130	760	—	—			YES	NO	—	?
54	F	72	313	9	360	105	510	108	520	—	—			YES	NO	NO	YES
48	F	82	210	—	—	100	585	130	660	130	810			YES	NO	YES	NO

- REASONS FOR DISCONTINUING THE TEST
a- MUSCULAR FATIGUE
b- SUBMAXIMAL HEART RATE
c- DECREASING OR STEADY-STATE OF THE HEART RATE
d- $\dot{V}O_2$ BEHAVIOUR

Although the implanted patients that achieve sinus rhythm during
exercise are closer to the normal group, we must underline that
these patients rarely achieved expected submaximal heart rate.
Moreover the rate changes during exercise, isn't proportional to
the increase of the load. So in valuing the criteria that
can be a guide in the conduction of an ergometric test, the heart
rate is not reliable.

When the heart rate doesn't increase from one work load to another in these patients (and we know that under this condition we have to
stop the test) we found the evaluation of the oxygen consumption useful in continuing the test. For this reason we carried out the test
in all patients with the oxygen consumption guide.

The reasons for interrupting the exercise test were the
same for all: muscular fatigue.

As we have already said, the pacemaker implanted patients
are able to have a physical activity which is apparently not
different from normal subjects, but functional adaptability at
different work loads is not the same.

In fact the oxygen consumption in the spontaneous and sinus
rhythm patients is respectively 82.5% and 86.7% against the
control group, while in paced rhythm patients it is clearly
lower (75.8%). This data confirms those of other authors (9).

The unfavourable condition of these patients in the latter
group emerges also from the analysis of the relationship between
ventilation and oxygen consumption. In fact the paced rhythm
patients need a higher level of ventilation in comparison to
the other two groups, in order to obtain equal oxygen consumption.
This condition is certainly unfavourable, knowing the relationship
between "excess ventilation" and possibility of metabolic
acidosis (12).

The measurement of maximum aerobic power has been introduced
as a clinical routine programme to evaluate the functional
condition of the cardiovascular system. The oxygen uptake gives
an indirect evaluation of the cardiac output. During the maximum
exercise there is a linear relationship between the maximum
oxygen uptake and the maximum cardiac output (13).

Because the pacemaker implanted patients have shown to
have a lower aerobic capacity in respect to the normal
subjects, there is no doubt that this must be referred to the
fact that the adaptability of the cardiac output is not
suitable to functional needs.

It is known that there are two ways to increase the cardiac output: increase the heart rate and increase the stroke volume (14). Both of these are possible in patients who achieved spontaneous rhythm, and especially in patients who achieved sinus rhythm; nevertheless we know that in these patients a limited adaptability of heart rate exists. The paced rhythm patients can utilize only the change of stroke volume to increase their cardiac output. For this reason in this group the increase of the oxygen pulse is significant, for it corresponds to the amount of the oxygen removed from the tissues by the blood ejected at each heart beat.

Although utilizing this hemodynamic adaptability, these patients are those with a lower oxygen consumption and consequently a lower cardiac output.

It follows that with regard to physical acitivity the ideal type of pacemaker would be the one that allows a proportional increase of the heart rate, namely the atrial synchronous pacer. With this type of pacemaker the paced rhythm patients could also reach functional levels similar to the other groups.

The functional evaluation of pacemaker implanted patients could offer, as perspective, the possibility of a physical reconditioning. To speak about rehabilitation in these patients is probably aleatory. As the paced patients can hardly use the physiological variation of heart rate, the highest chance derives from the change that physical training determines at peripheral levels.

SUMMARY

During the physical acitivity the functional condition of the cardiovascular system needs an increased heart rate that the normal pacemaker can't give. It is for this reason that the implanted patient has a different hemodynamic behaviour, and it is necessary to know the guiding criteria in the programme of an ergometric test, and to establish the usefulness of the findings in order to evaluate his physical capacity.

For these reasons we studied 28 pacemaker implanted patients. The functional evaluation of the physical capacity had been made with discontinuous cycle ergometer test. 15 subjects had been selected as a control group. The oxygen consumption, the ECG and the blood pressure were recorded.

During the exercises 5 patients remained paced at the proper rate of the pacemaker. The heart rate increased in 9 patients as a result of a spontaneous rhythm. In the remaining 14

patients sinus rhythm was restored. There wasn't any statistical
difference between all groups in respect of work load. The
group of patients with paced rhythm during exercise had lower
aerobic capacity compared to the control group and the other
two groups.

The paced rhythm patients had a O_2P of 12.21 ± 3 SD; the
spontaneous rhythm patients 9.9 ± 2.9 SD; sinus rhythm patients
8.34 ± 2.1 SD; control group 7.8 ± 1.5 SD. A significant difference
exists in comparing the three groups of patients ($p<0.05$).
There is a high level of difference ($p<0.001$) between paced
rhythm patients and control group. There is no significant
difference between sinus rhythm group and control, while there
is a significant difference between spontaneous rhythm and
control ($p<0.05$).

In the control group the higher oxygen consumption
corresponds to lower oxygen pulse. This characteristic has a
tendency to invert if one observes our groups with sinus rhythm,
spontaneous rhythm or paced rhythm.

In our research we have taken into account the relationship
between ventilation and oxygen consumption. The paced rhythm
patients show a line with higher slope in respect to all the other
groups; they need more ventilation for the same oxygen
consumption.

Because the pacemaker implanted patients have shown to
have a lower aerobic capacity in respect to the normal subjects,
there is no doubt that this must be referred to the fact that
the adaptability of the cardiac output is not suitable to
functional needs.

To speak about physical rehabilitation in these patients is
probably aleatory.

As the paced patient can hardly use the physiological
varation of the heart rate the highest chance derives from the
change that physical training determines at peripheral level.

References

1. E. Sowton: Haemodynamic studies in patients with artificial
    pacemaker. Brit.Heart J. 26:737 (1964).
2. I. N. Segel, W. A. Hudson, P. Harris, J. M. Bishop: The
    circulatory effects of electrically induced changes in
    ventricular rate at rest and during exercise in complete heart
    block. J. Clin.Invest. 43:1541 (1964).

3. P. Samet, C. Castillo, W. H. Bernestein, S. Levine:
    Significance of the atrial contribution to ventricular
    pacing. Am.J.Cardiol. 15:195 (1965).

4. A. Benchimol, J. G. Ellis, E. G. Diamond: Hemodynamic
    consequences of atrial and ventricular pacing in patients
    with normal and abnormal hearts. Effect of exercise at fixed
    atrial and ventricular rate. Am.J.Med. 39:911 (1965).

5. R. A. Carleton, R. W. Sessions, J. S. Graettinger: Cardiac
    pacemakers: clinical and physiological studies. Med.Clin.
    N.Amer. 50:325 (1966).

6. P. Samet, C. Castillo, W. H. Bernestein: Hemodynamic
    consequences of sequential atrioventricular pacing.
    Subjects with normal hearts. Am.J.Cardiol.21:207 (1968).

7. A. Raineri, M. Traina, G. Indovina, A. Castello, P. Assennato,
    L. Messina: L'impedenza toracica nella sorveglianza dei
    pazienti ricoverati in Unità Coronarica. Boll.Soc.Ital.
    Cardiol. 22:1859 (1977).

8. V. Rulli, P. Signoretti, A. Nardelli, P. Rossi: Valutazione
    della capacità funzionale in soggetti portatori di
    elettrostimolatori artificiali. Giorn.Ital.Card. 1:26 (1971).

9. H. Ikeda, N. Koga, F. Katayama, K. Ohishi, H. Toshima,
    N. Kimura: Functional capacity of pacemaker implanted patients.
    Proceedings of the 5th International Symposium, Tokya (1976)
    page 304.

10. A. Holmgran, P. Karlberg, B. Pernow: Circulatory adaptation
    at rest and during muscular work in patients with complete
    heart block. Acta med.Scandanav. 164:119 (1959).

11. D. Ikkos, J. Hanson: Response to exercise in congenital
    complete atrioventricular block. Circulation 22:583 (1960).

12. S. N. Koyal, B. J. Wipp, D. Huntsman, G. A. Bray, K. Wasserman:
    Ventilatory responses to the metabolic acidosis of treadmill
    and cycle ergometry. J.Appl.Phys. 40:864 (1976).

13. K. L. Andersen, R. J. Shephard, H. Denolin, E. Varnauskas,
    R. Masironi, Fundamentals of exercise testing. World
    Health Organization (1971); page 24-26.

14. S. F. Vatner, M. Pagani: Adattamenti cardiovascolari
    all'attività fisica: emodinamica e meccanismi. Progressi
    in Patol.Cardiov. 2:155 (1978).

ECHOCARDIOGRAPHY IN CARDIAC FUNCTIONAL EVALUATION AND

REHABILITATION

S. Sandric

Instituto di Patologia Medica
Università Cattolica, Roma
Italy

Much of the recent interest in echocardiography has been stimulated by reports that this technique can be used to evaluate left ventricular function (anatomy and performance).

X-ray contrast angiography, radionuclide angiography, derivation of systolic time intervals and clinical assessment of left ventricular function are all imperfect and cumbersome means of deriving parameters of cardiac function.

There is much controversy about the significance, sensitivity, and purity of these measurement in helping us assess the state of the myocardium in a given patients. At the present time, echocardiography cannot solve this problem but it can provide further data for analysis.

The recent advent of echocardiography has provided an atraumatic technique which has been demonstrated to be capable of reliable evaluating several aspects of cardiac anatomy and performance.

Echochardiography provides accurate measurements of left ventricular cavitary size, wall thickness, wall motion, end-systolic and end-diastolic left ventricular volumes.

Several investigators proved that, mean rate of circumferential fibre shortening correlate well with other indices of myocardial contractility and a good correlation also has been demonstrated between mean Vcf estimated angiographically and that estimated echocardiographically.

Feigenbaum showed a good correlation between the volume

estimated by echocardiography and volumes estimated by left
ventricular angiography (4).

Therefore, echocardiography has been proposed as an alternative
mean to cardiac catheterization in assessing cardiac anatomy,
volumes, ventricular size, and in estimating left ventricular
compliance because of distinct advantage of being a noninvasive
atraumatic method lending itself readily to serial measurements.

There are several ways in which one can examine portion of
the left ventricule. Standardized measurement of cyclic change
in left ventricular diameter is the row data processed to assess
the integrity of the myocardium. Standardization is aided by
using end-diastolic and end-systolic dimensions of the left
ventricular cavity. (Fig. 1).

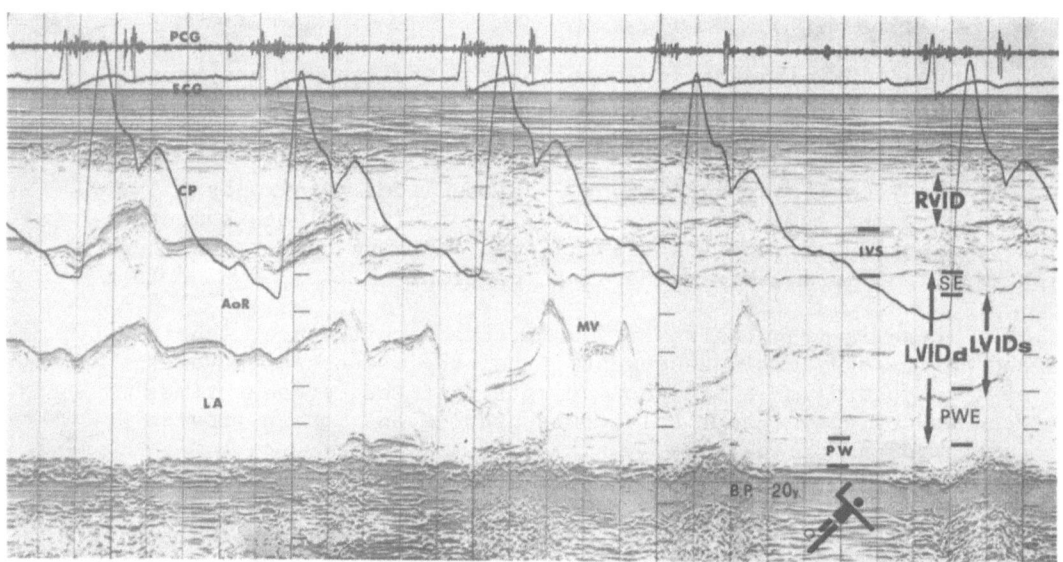

Fig. 1.   An M-mode echocardiogram with continuous recording from
          a normal subject. PCG = Phonocardiogram; ECG =
          Electrocardiogram; CP = Carotid pulse; AoR = Aortic root;
          LA = Left antrium; MV = Mitral valve; IVS = Interventricular
          septum; PW = Posterior wall; PWE = Posterior wall
          excursion; SE = Septal excursion; LCIDd = Left ventricular
          end-diastolic dimension; VLIDs = Left ventricular end-
          systolic dimension; RVID = Right ventricular internal
          dimension.

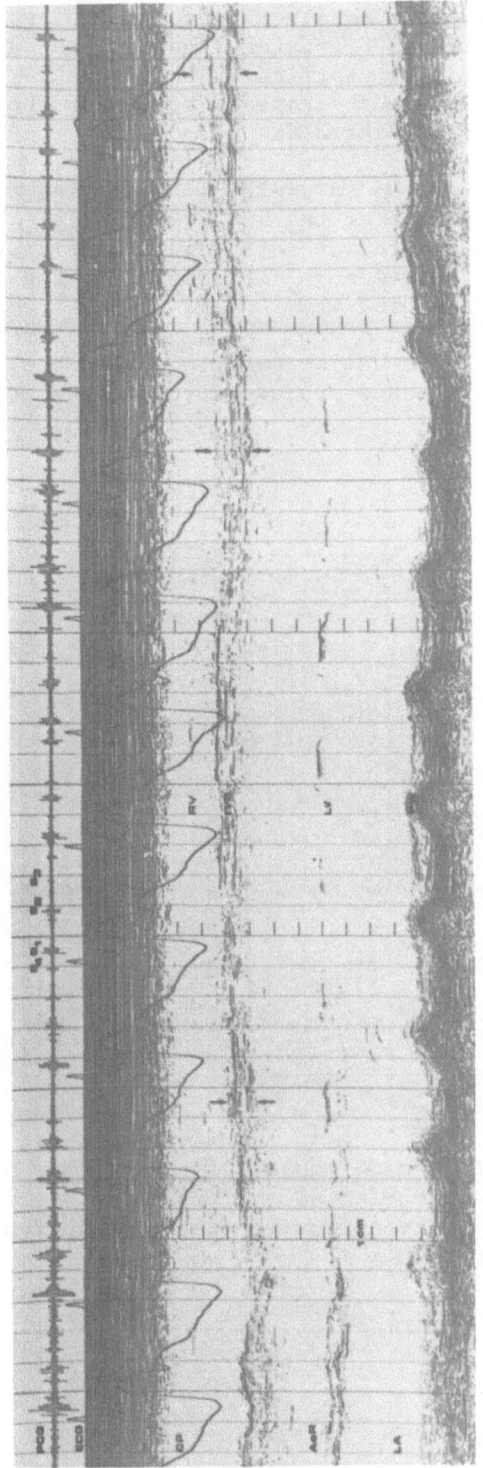

Figure 2. M-mode linear scan echocardiogram recording from a patient with left ventricular aneurysm. Arrows indicate changes in thickness, motion and appearance of adjacent segments of septum.

It is possible merely to measure the amplitude of motion
of cardiac walls with greater accuracy than any other technique,
even including left ventricular angiography. Also it is
possible to measure the rate of motion of the wall segment
during systole or diastole.

The examination is useful in detecting akynetic or
diskynetic segments of the left ventricule. It may even by able to
quantitate the degree of left ventricular disfunction. Very
accurate is measurement of the amount of the cardiac wall during
systole and diastole.

Scar tissue could be detected by echocardiography having a
higher density, hence produce more intense echoes (Fig. 2).

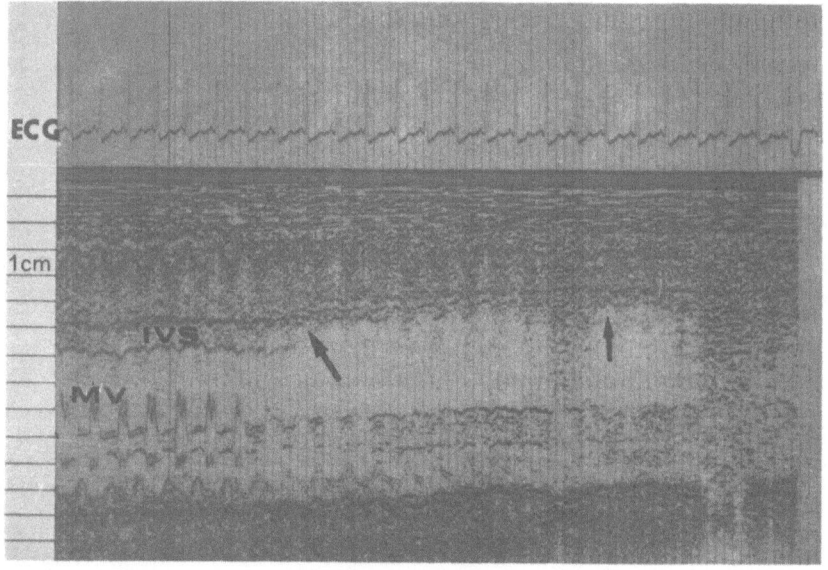

Figure 3.   An M-mode echocardiogram from a patient with a large
             antero-septal myocardial infarction. Thickening of
             interventricular septum is increased. (arrows).

The method also provides information concerning over-all shape of the left ventricle.

The technique is useful in the detection of left ventircular aneurysm, as is showed in Fig. 3.

The echocardiogram is a superb tool in identifying mobile and fixed intracardiac masses. Masses in cardiac cavity generally produce intense echoes with a peculiar shaggy appearance attached to the ventricular wall.

Fig. 4 shows a left ventricular thrombi attached to the posterior left ventricular wall in a patient with acute myocardial infarction.

One can obtain information about left ventricular performance by looking at other parts of the echocardiogram besides left ventricular hemodynamics. There is evidence that the pattern of mitral valve motion may reflect changes in left ventricular diastolic pressure.

In patients who have an elevated left ventricular end-diastolic pressure because of poor ventricular compliance and an elevated atrial component, there is a distortion of the mitral valve echo. Closure is altered in a predictable way so that one can tell from the echocardiogram of mitral valve when the left ventricular end-diastolic pressure is markedly elevated (Fig. 5).

Aortic valve motion may also reflect flow across the aortic valve. In patients with low cardiac output, the aortic valve gradually closes during systole (Fig. 4). It has been noted that the patient with severe or even moderate IHSS, there may have a mid-systolic closure of the aortic valve at blood flow into the aorta due to the obstruction.

Some study suggests that there even may be a correlation between amplitude and duration of aortic valve separation and aortic valve flow.

The number of echocardiographic measurements which may be useful in finding ventricular performance seems to be increasing.

Recently there has been interest in estimating blood flow velocity in man noninvasively by detecting the Doppler frequency shift of a beam of transmitted ultrasound.

In order to measure the angle of the ultrasound beam relative to the flowing stream of blood, a Doppler velocimeter

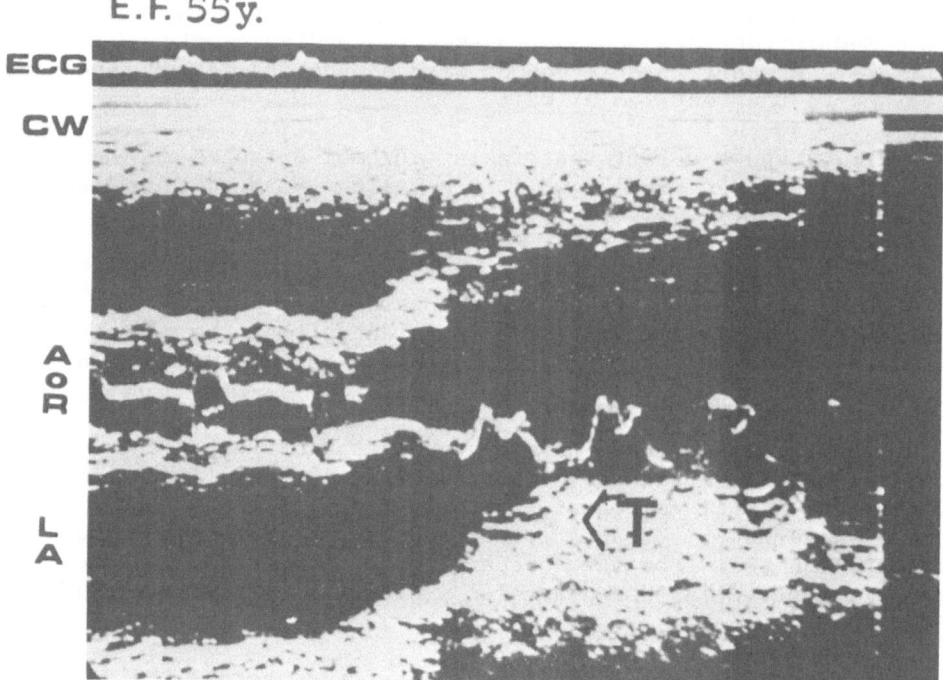

Fig. 4. Sector scan recording of the left ventricle showing (T)
         a mass of dense echoes within the left ventricular
         cavity attached to the posterior wall which is markedly
         hypoactive and takes origin in the left atrium.

has been combined with a two-dimensional imagining system that
allows the blood vessel to be imaged at the same time that the
Doppler sample volume is superimposed on the image.

    This directional capability may be of limited use in the
pulmonary artery but should be particularly helpful when
measuring blood flow in the aorta and inside the heart where
both forward and backward flow might be expected.

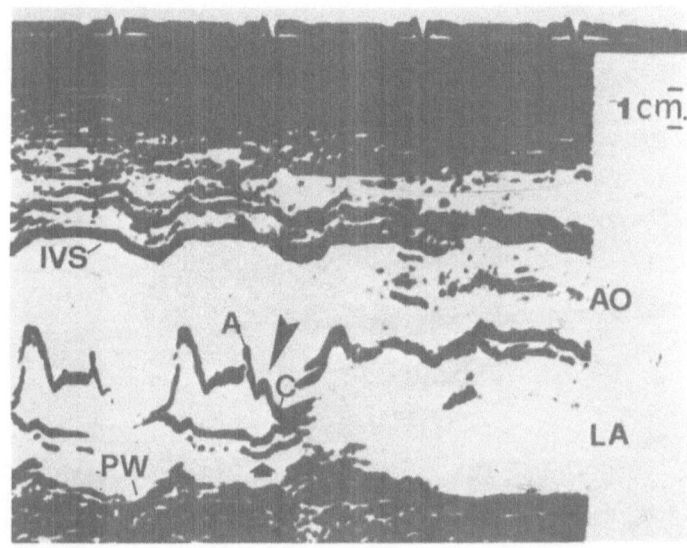

Fig. 5.   Abnormal echocardiogram showing a thin (PW) scarred
          and dyskinetic posterior wall in a patient with myocardial
          infarction of posterior wall. Arrow indicated a
          markedly increased atrial component; anterior movement
          of anterior mitral leaflet at the end-diastole,
          which reflects changes in left ventricular end-
          diastolic pressure.

     It is hoped that this approach will eventually allow the
noninvasive measurement of volume blood flow in man.

     Echocardiography can currently provide considerable
information concerning left ventricular function at rest and
during exercise.

     Using exercise echocardiography (Fig. 6) it is possible to
evaluate directly the influence of exercise training upon left
ventricular intracavitary size, wall thickness and contractile
pattern, in normal subjects, well trained athletes and patients
with ischemic heart disease.

     The greatest limitation of this technique is the difficulty
in obtaining high quality echocardiograms during exercise.

     From a practical point of view, moreover, reproducible
echocardiograms during exercise in a sitting position are very
difficult to record. Much better data could be obtained from
echocardiograms recorded in supine position.

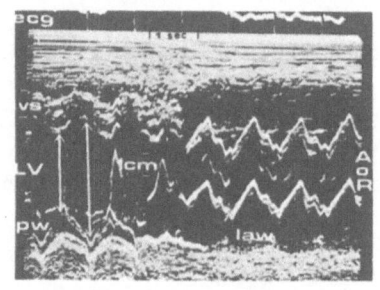

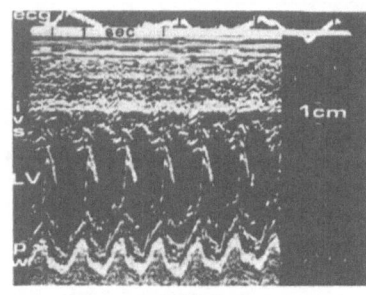

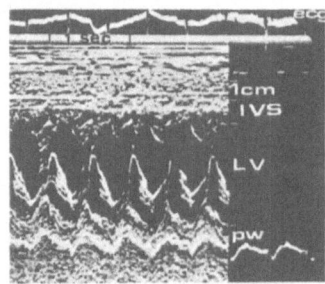

Fig. 6. Pre and during exercise training echocardiogram, showing
         changes in thickness, motion and internal dimensions,
         from a well trained athlete.

Unequivocal evidence of a training effect was observed
following the physical conditioning in normal subjects and
well trained athletes (1,2,9,10).

The results of echocardiographic studies indicated that
significant alterations in cardiac anatomy were induced by
physical conditioning.

The changes in left ventricular wall thickness, cardiac
internal dimensions and ventricular performance during the
exercise training were observed.

Although, echocardiographic data clearly demonstrate that
exercise training is capable of inducing definite alterations
in cardiac structure and function, the precise biologic
significane of these changes cannot be determined at present.

In humans, the resting echocardiogram in patients without previous infarction is a poor predictor of the presence of coronary disease. (3).

Echocardiograms have been recorded during angina produced by handgrip-stress and have demonstrated reduced wall motion amplitude, ejection fraction and Vcf.

Unfortunately, these abnormalities have only been seen in some patients, and all of them had high grade coronary disease (6).

There are several advantages of exercise echocardiography in the evaluation of patients with ischemic heart disease. Echocardiography is the only technique widely available for measuring dynamic changes in wall thickness in different regions of the heart.

In the presence of resting regional hypokinesis, echocardiography during exercise might detect improvement in regional function and localize a potentially viable wall segment similar to the effect of intervention-ventriculography.

With the increasing number of good investigators entering the field and with many potential technical and engineering improvements get to be explored, there is every reason to believe that some of this present limitation will be eliminated and that echocardiography will become one of the best methods available for judging left ventricular performance.

References

1. P. Bubenheimer, H. Roskamm, L. Samek and H. J. Schmeisser. Echocardiographie zur Beurteilung der Arbeitsweise des linken Ventrikels unter dynamischer körperlicher Belastung. Sportarzt u. Sportmedizin 28:345 (1977).
2. A. N. De Maria, A. Neumann, G. Lee, W. Fowler and D. Mason. Alteration in ventricular mass and performance induced by exercise training in man evaluated by echocardiography. Circulation 57:237 (1978).
3. A. C. Dortmer, R. L. De Joseph, R. A. Schiroff and R. Zelis. Echocardiographic predictors of coronary artery disease. Clin. Res. 24:215 A (1976) (abstr.).
4. H.Feigenbaum. Echocardiography. 11° Ed. Philadelphia, Lea and Febiger, (1976).
5. J. M. Griffith and W. Henry. An ultrasound system for combined cardiac imaging and Doppler blood flow measurement in men. Circulation 57:925 (1978).
6. W. Klein, P. Pavek. Belastungechokardiographie bei koronares herzkrankheit (Exercise echocardiography in

coronary heart disease). Z. Kardiol. 66:112 (1977).

7. S. J. Mason, J. L. Weiss, M. L. Weisfeldt, J. B. Garrison
    and J. Fortuin. Exercise echocardiography; detection of
    wall motion abnormalities during ischemia. Circulation
    59:50 (1979).

8. S. Rasmussen, B. C. Corya, H. Feigenbaum and S. B. Knoebel.
    Detection of myocardial scar tissue by M—mode echocardiography.
    Circulation 57:230 (1978).

9. R. Rost, W. Hollmann, H. Gerhardus, H. Philippi. Die
    Anwendung der Echocardiographie in der Sportmedizin.
    Sportarzt und Sportmedizin, 28:103 (1977).

10. S. Sandric, P. Zeppilli, G. Assorgi, F. Cecchetti and
    G. Piovana. Echocardiographic assessment of left ventricular
    performance in highly trained rowers during and after
    exhaustive work. International Conference on sports
    Cardiology, Rome April 1978.

RESTING AND EXERCISE SYSTOLIC TIME INTERVALS

P. Assennato, E. Hoffmann, and A. Raineri

Cattedra di Fisiopatologia Cardiovascolare
Università di Palermo
Italy

The measurement of Systolic Time Intervals (STI), for the indirect assessment of ventricular function, has become one of the established "non-invasive" techniques of clinical cardiology. (1,2).

Easy to apply, like all non-invasive techniques the STI have the advantage that multiple observations can be performed.

This study was designed to evaluate if measurements of STI after exercise are potentially of more value than measurements at rest.

MATERIAL AND METHODS

Twenty-four male subjects, aged 35 to 55 (average 45 years) who had a well documented episode of myocardial infarction were studied three months after the acute stage. At the time of the study all these subjects were asymptomatic, with no clinical signs of heart failure.

Thirty-nine healthy subjects, aged 18 to 55 (average 38 years) were studied as a control group.

Systolic Time Intervals were determined at fast, in the morning in supine position, at rest and four minutes after a submaximal exertion test conducted with a bicycle ergometer. All heart patients had discontinued therapy a week before being included in this study.

Simultaneous indirect carotid artery pulse tracings, phono-cardiograms, and electrocardiograms, were recorded by an

Elema-Schönander Mingograf 34 recording system at a paper speed of 100 mm/sec.

Systolic Time Intervals included total electromechanic systol (QA_2), left ventricular ejection time (LVET), the pre-ejection period (PEP), and PEP/LVET ratio, determined in a manner previously described by Weissler. (3). All intervals were determined as the average measurement of at least six consecutive beats, and were corrected for the heart rate using regression lines, computed before and after exercise on a control group of 39 healthy subjects.

Statistical analyses were performed by the Student's method and by the analysis of the linear regression, to study the relationship between Systolic Time Indexes and heart rate.

QA_2 and LVET values in coronary patients were corrected with regard to the heart rate using the values of the regression lines obtained in normal subjects before and after exercise. Such a correction was not carried out with regard to PEP, due to the lack of relationship between PEP and heart rate, before and after exercise ($r=0.44$ and $r=0.20$ respectively).

RESULTS

The comparison between regression lines of LVET before and after exercise in healthy subjects, does not show any difference with the exception of the intercept, which is moderately higher after exercise than at rest (Fig. 1); the regression lines of QA_2 before and after exercise, show a different trend, both for the intercept and for the slope. Even if not very high a significant correlation exists between LVET, QA_2 and heart rate.

The correction factors utilized were those concerning the 39 normal subjects, before and after exercise, and they were for QA_2 2.11 at rest and 1.85 after exercise; for LVET 1.62 at rest and 1.67 after exercise.

The behaviour of the electromechanic systole index (QA_2I) in our subjects (FIg. 2) shows a difference in the resting values of healthy individuals and heart patients, the latter group showing higher values which differ statistically ($p<0.02$) from those of the healthy subjects. After exercise QA_2I shows a shortening of the resting values, which is significant in the heart patients only ($p<0.01$).

Although the left ventricular ejection time index (LVETI) values show no significant difference between the two groups, either before or after exercise, increased values of LVETI have been noticed among the subjects of the same groups after exercise.

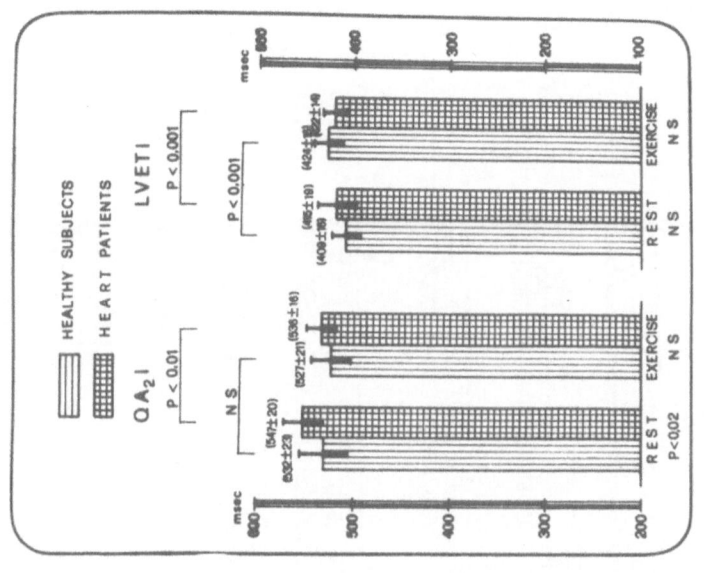
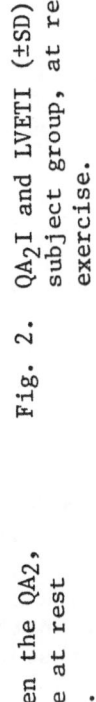

Fig. 2. QA₂I and LVETI (±SD) mean in each subject group, at rest and after exercise.

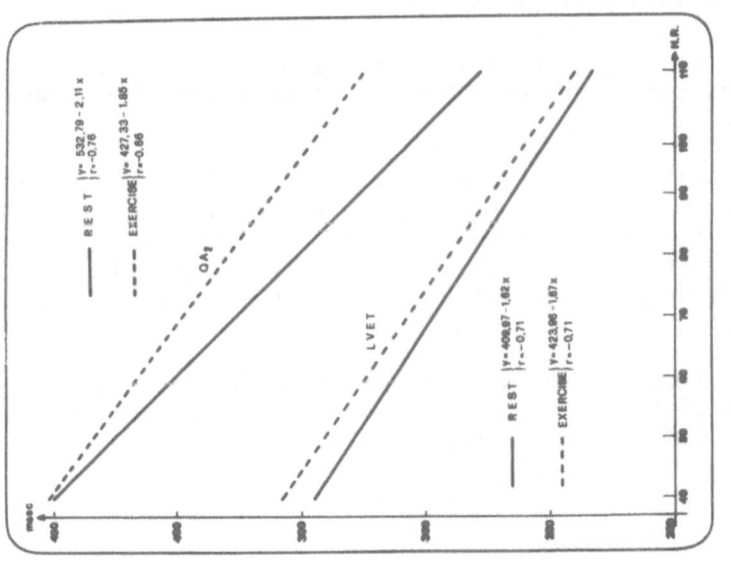

Fig. 1. Relationship between the QA2, LVET and heart rate at rest and after exercise.

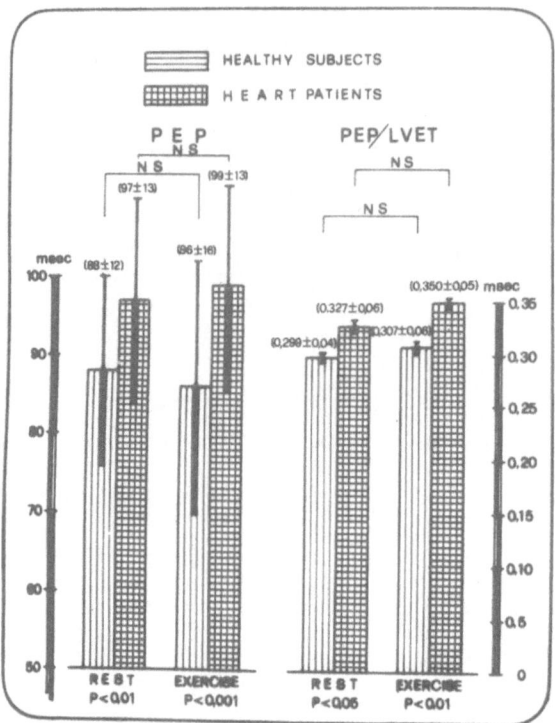

Fig. 3.   PEP and PEP/LVET ratio (±SD) mean in each subject group, at
          rest and after exercise.

     The values of the pre-ejection period (PEP) and PEP-LVET
ratio in the two groups of subjects, at rest and after exercise
are presented in Fig. 3.

     Heart patients show at rest longer pre-ejection period than
healthy subjects. This difference is statistically significant
(p<0.01). After exercise this difference becomes more evident
(p<0.001); there is a non-significant shortening of PEP in healthy
individuals, and a non-significant lengthening in patients with
infarction.

     PEP/LVET ratio and PEP behaviour are similar. In fact the
rest values of this index are higher in the heart subject than in
normal (p<0.05). After exercise the difference between the two
groups increases (p<0.01).

Discussion

     According to what has been reported in the literature,
Systolic Time Intervals were measured four minutes after
exercise. Lewis has determined Systolic Time Intervals at

rest and 2, 4, 6, 10 minutes after exercise, showing that 4 minutes
after exterion is the best point in time to distinguish normal
subjects from heart patients; there is a return to resting blood
pressure values on the 4th minute of the recovery phase, while
the influence of heart rate is less evident. (2-4).

The choosing of the measurement time is a very relevant
factor in evaluating the result of Systolic Time Intervals
obtained after exercise in different studies. This many explain
the differences reported in the literature up to date, but type
of exertion loads, measurement time, and posture may influence
in many ways the recording of STI. (5).

In our study, the lengthening of the resting QA_2I, seems to
show that the electromechanic systole is longer in patients
with myocardial infarction than in normal subjects.

While some AAs have not noticed significant changes in
resting QA_2I values in normal subjects as compared with heart
patients, our observations are in agreement with those of Lauwers
et al., who believe the lengthening of QA_2I to be the result of
changes in the time of the isovolumetric contraction. (6). In
point of fact, QA_2I consists of the summation of more intervals,
and its interpretation may be ambiguous if considered as a single
interval, without taking into consideration its components.

Using apex-cardiography, Wilhelmsen showed a lengthening of
the electromechanical interval from the beginning of the QRS
complex to the systolic upstroke of the apex-cardiogram, in
infarct patients (7).

After exercise in both our groups, the electromechanic
systole shows a shortening, which is significant only in patients
with myocardial infarction. The cause of this phenomenon is likely
to be seen in the increase of circulating catecholamines (8). In
fact the QA_2I is remarkably decreased in all those conditions
where a high rate of blood catecholamines is present (thyrotoxicosis,
congestive heart failure) (10,11). The pattern of this interval
after exercise, suggests marked adrenergic hyperactivity in the
coronary patient. As known, the administration of propanolol after
exercise causes a significant lengthening of QA_2I in subjects
with coronary affections. Consistently, Lewis thinks that the
QA_2I, can be soundly used as an index of adrenergic hyperactivity
in coronary patients (9).

The LVETI values obtained in the course of our research do
not show significant changes in the healthy subjects when compared
with patients with myocardial infarction. On the contrary, both
groups respond to effort by lengthening the values of LVETI.

LVETI is thought to depend prevalently on the stroke volume which, in turn, depends on different factors such as metabolic requirements, after loads, teledyastolic volume, myocardial contractility (12,13). The stroke volume increases, which raise the extend of fiber shortening, cause a lengthening of LVETI (14), while positive inotropic agents which cause an increase of the velocity of fiber shortening, are responsible for the decrease of LVETI (15). The velocity and extend of fiber shortening play a relevant role in influencing LVETI values. The velocity of fiber shortening during the left ventricular failure ejection phase is diminished; this condition should in theory produce a lengthening of LVETI (16). Nevertheless, the extend of fiber shortening is reduced, and this should tend to shorten LVETI. However, the latter condition usually prevails in the left ventricular failure, thus resulting in a shortening of LVETI.

Unlike PEP, which goes the opposite way, positive and negative inotropic agents both shorten LVETI (15, 17-19); the positive agents by increasing velocity of fiber shortening, and the negative agents by diminishing the extent.

The factors which influence LVETI behaviour are multifarious and often opposing, and this makes it difficult to understand the meaning of LVETI lengthening observed by us in normal subjects, after submaximal effort. It is likely that LVETI increase observed in our series may be referred to the increased venour return, when getting from orthostatic to supine position after exercise.

The shortening found in our study is not in agreement with the values obtained by some AAs (Lewis, Pouget) (4,20), who have noticed a shortening, or no change, in the value of LVETI, while it agrees with those of McConahay (21). Cardus, on the other hand, has noticed differing values in normal subjects, according to the age range, of the group examined; young people showed a shortening during exercise, while older (but not elderly) individuals showed a relative lengthening of LVETI, which could be justified by a valid, but less vigourous, myocardial contraction (22). All these AAs, on the other hand, have been using a methodology differing, either in the type and degree of exercise, or in the time of intervals monitoring.

Patients with infarction have shown a pattern similar to that of the control group, and no significant changes. This is difficult to understand. Other AAs (McConahay), in agreement with our result, have found a lengthening of LVETI values, in both healthy and heart subjects. These results contradict those of Pouget and Lewis, who obtained after exercise a shortening of LVETI in healthy subjects and a lengthening of LVETI in coronary

patients, ascribing to this parameter considerable importance in
separating the healthy subjects from heart patients.

The affinity of LVETI values between the two groups in our
series is possible to be seen in the fact that our patients were
asymptomatic and in satisfactory cardiac compensation.

PEP has proved to be a very sensitive index in distinguishing
healthy people from patients with myocardial infarction. In fact
the values at rest and after exercise, noticed in our series, are
significantly higher than those seen in normal subjects. The
PEP most conditioning haemodynamic factors are the LVEDP, the
velocity of the left ventricular pressure rising (LVdp/dt), the
aortic dyastolic pressure (23,24). Thus, the PEP lengthening is
the result of the left ventricular performance as a whole, which
cannot be ascribed to single factors, such as the diminished
contractility (3). Other variables should be taken into account,
such as volume, ventricular mass, synergy,. Therefore, PEP
is a measure of the ventricular performance as a whole during
the isovolumetric phase. Consequently, the PEP lengthening could
be the result of a diminished left ventricular performance, due
to the lack of response to effort stimuli.

The behaviour of PEP in normal subjects coincides with already
published results, in the sense of a shortening of this index
after effort, although not all the AAs are in agreement as far as
coronary patients are concerned (20, 21). Nevertheless, many of
these AAs have investigated patients with angina pectoris, rather
than with asymptomatic myocardial infarction.

Also the ratio PEP/LVET may be considered as a parameter,
which shows significantly differing values in healthy people and
in infarcted patients at rest and after exercise. As the PEP/LVET
shows no correlation with heart rate, its variations offer the
advantage of showing the changes in both basic intervals, PEP
and LVET, and thus reveal the presence of anomalies, when neither
of the two indexes is clearly abnormal (25). This relationship
has been correlated to the cardiac index, and, particularly, to
the left ventricular ejection fraction as determined by
quantitative angiography (26).

Our basic STI results do not differ from those usually
reported in the literature (23). Substantial differences have
been on the contrary, noticed in the after exercise results.

This disagreement may be explained by differing methodologies
and degree of exercise, differing time and mode of intervals
measuring, use of different correcting factors and selection of
subjects to be studied (age, disease, etc.). All these factors
may produce changes in the STI response to exercise.

Considering the type of patients included in our series and the methodology adopted, PEP and PET/LVET, represent the systolic intervals, which proved to be most valuable in separating healthy people from patients with myocardial infarction.

Nevertheless, one has to proceed cautiously in evaluating the results, for many variables may change them.

The possibility of normaly PEP/LVET values in acute stage of myocardial infarction shows that these indexes "per se" cannot be held to have absolute value in evaluating the left ventricular performance (27), which needs the support of further investigations (invasive and non-invasive) to allow a reliable definition of the stage of a coronary affection.

References

1. R. P. Lewis, S. E. Rittgers, W. F. Forester, H. Boudoulas: A critical review of the Systolic Time Intervals, Circulation 56::146 (1977).
2. R. P. Lewis, H. Boudoulas, T. G. Welch, W. F. Forester: Usefulness of Systolic Time Intervals in coronary artery disease. Am. J. Cardiol, 37:787 (1976).
3. A. M. Weissler: Cardiologia non invasiva, Il Pensiero Scientifico Editore (1977) pp.258-260.
4. R.P.Lewis, D. G. Marsh, J. A. Sherman, W. F. Forester, S. F. Schaal: Enhanced diagnostic power of exercise testing for myocardial ischemia by addition of post-exercise left ventricular ejection time. Am. J. Cardiol, 39:707 (1977).
5. P. S. Nandi, D. H. Spodick: Recovery from exercise at varying work loads. Time course of responses of heart rate and Systolic Intervals. Br. Heart J., 39:958 (1977).
6. M. Leisse, K. Imschoot, P. Lauwers, C. Mertens: Comparison du pouls carotidien de suject normaux et coronarieus. Arch. mal coeur, 69:296 (1976).
7. L. Wilhelmsen: The value of systolic and diastolic time intervals. Br. Heart J., 40:256 (1978)
8. C. Valori, M. Thomas, J. Shillingford: Free noradrenaline and adrenaline excretion in relation to clinical syndromes following myocardial infarction. Am. J. Cardiol., 20:605 (1967).
9. R. P. Lewis, H. Boudoulas, W. F. Forester et al.: Shortening of electromechanical systole as a manifestation of excessive adrenergic stimulation in acute myocardial infarction. Circulation 46:856 (1972).
10. R. Hegglin: What is the significance of a shortened systole, Cardiologia, 48:71 (1966).
11. H. P. Krayenbuhl, H. Buble, H. Cander, R. Hegglin: Die dauer des intervalls Q-11 herzton (elektromechanische systole) beim herzgesundeu, sportler, herzinsuffizienter und hyperthyreotiker. Helv.med. Acta. 32: suppl.45, 34 (1965).

12. A. M. Weissler, R. G. Peeler, W. H. Rohell: Relationship between left ventricular ejection time, stroke volume, and heart rate in normal individuals and patients with cardiovascular disease. Amer. Heart J. 62:367 (1961).

13. E. Braunwald, J. Rossi, E. H. Sonnenblick: Mechanism of contraction of the normal and failing heart. Little Brown, Boston (1967), pp.58.

14. A. M. Weissler, C. D. Scheonfeld: Effect of digitalis on systolic time intervals in heart failure. Am.J. Med. Sci. 259:4 (1970).

15. S. H. Salzman, S. Wolfson, B. Jackson, E. Scheeter: Epinephrine infusion in man. Standardization, normal response, and abnormal response in idiopatic hypertrophic subaortic stenosis. Circulation 43:137 (1971).

16. J. H. Gault, J. Ross Jr., E. Braunwald: Contractile state of the left ventricle in man. Circ. Res. 22:(4), 451 (1968).

17. W. S. Harris, C. D. Schoenfeld, R. H. Brooks, A. M. Weissler: Effect of beta adrenergic blockade on the haemodynamic responses to epinephrine in man. Am. J. Cardiol. 17:484 (1966).

18. W. S. Harris, C. D. Schoenfeld, A. M. Weissler: Effect of adrenergic receptor activation and blockade on the systolic pre-ejection period, heart rate and arterial pressure in man. J. Clin. Invest. 46:1704 (1967).

19. D. Hunt, G. Sloman, R. M. Clark, G. Hoffmann: Effects of beta-adrenergic blockade on the systolic time intervals. Am..J.Med.Sci. 259:97 (1970).

20. J. M. Pouget, W. S. Harris, B. R. Mayron: Abnormal responses of the systolic time interval to exercise in patients with angina pectoris. Circulation 43:289 (1971).

21. D. R. McConahay, M. Carrol, M. C. Martin, M. Cheitlin: Resting and exercise systolic time intervals. Correlation with ventricular performance in patients with coronary artery disease. Circulation 45:592 (1972).

22. D. Cardus, L. Vera: Systolic Time Intervals at rest and during exercise. Cardiology 59:133 (1974).

23. C. E. Martin, J. A. Shaver, M. E. Thompson: Direct correlation of external systolic time intervals with internal indices of ventricular function in man. Circulation 44:419 (1971).

24. C. C. Metzger, C. B. Chough, F. W. Kroets: True isovolumic contraction time: Its correlation with two external indexes of ventricular performance. Am. J. Cardiol. 25:434 (1970).

25. A. M. Weissler, W. S. Harris, C. D. Scheonfeld: Bedside technics for the evaluation of ventricular function in man. Am.J. Cardiol. 23:577 (1969).

26. C. L. Garrad Jr., A. M. Weissler, H. T. Dodge: The relation-
    ship of alterations in systolic time intervals to ejection
    fraction in patients with cardiac disease. Circulation
    42:455 (1970).
27. B. W. Rama, N. H. Myers, A. G. Wallace et al.: Haemodynamic
    findings in 123 patients with acute myocardial infarction
    on admission. Circulation 42:567 (1970).

VALUE OF SYSTOLIC AND DIASTOLIC TIME INTERVALS

Lars Wilhelmsen, John Wikstrand, Göran Berglund,
and Ingemar Wallentin

Department of Medicine
Östra Hospital and the Department of Clinical Physiology
Sahlgrenska Hospital
Göteborg
Sweden

Non-invasively derived systolic time intervals for assessment of left ventricular function such as the left ventricular ejection time(LVET) and the pre-ejection period (PEP) have been extensively studied. PEP comprises the isovolumetric contraction time (ICT) and the interval from the beginning of depolarisation to the start of the systolic contraction, i.e. the electromechanical interval (EMI); it has been pointed out that the ICT should provide a better measure of left ventricular function than the PEP (12).

Prolongation of the PEP and shortening of the LVET with consequent prolongation of the PEP/LVET ratio have been ascribed to impaired contractility of the left ventricle. These changes in PEP and LVET have also been found to correlate well with contractility and measures of pump function (8, 2). Despite this, many authors doubted the value of the systolic time intervals (10, 16).

Several authors have used apex cardiography to measure the interval between the aortic component of the second heart sound (A_2) and the O-point in the apex cardiogram in order to study isovolumetric relaxation (21, 3, 13). Transducers with short low frequency time constants have often been used. These transducers, however, shorten the A_2O interval and tend to smooth out differences between a prolonged and a normal A_2O interval (11, 24).

Most of the above mentioned studies were carried out in small selected groups of hospital patients. The aim of the present study was to investigate the value of non-invasively registered time intervals in representative groups of untreated hypertensives and post-infarction patients, and to establish the normal limits for these intervals in 50-year-old men (30).

GROUPS STUDIED

All subjects of a random population sample of 50-year-old men in Göteborg, Sweden (32) with untreated essential hypertension group (n=35). Essential hypertension was defined by casual blood pressure above 175 mmHg systolic or 115 mmHg diastolic on two separate occasions and a negative diagnostic examination for secondary hypertension (31).

A reference group (n=73) with casual blood pressure below 175 mmHg systolic and 115 mmHg diastolic was obtained from the same population by drawing a 10 per cent subsample at random. The infarct group (n=67) consisted of men living in Göteborg, born between 1916 and 1924, who suffered a hospital verified myocardial infarction during a 12-month period (15 July 1972 to 14 July 1973) and survived for at least 3 months. The mean age for the infarct group was 53½ years (range 48 to 57). Fifty-nine patients had primary infarcts and 8 patients suffered from reinfarction. The non-invasive investigations were carried out in a randomised half of the reference group (n=36) and of the hypertension group (n=19) and all infarct patients (n=67).

METHODS

Conventional electrocardiograms, carotid pulse tracings, apex cardiograms, phonocardiograms, and resting blood pressures were all recorded on a direct writing ink-jet 7-channel mingograph (EM 81, Siemens-Elema AB, Sweden) with a linear frequency response from 0 to 500 Hz and 30 per cent amplitude reduction at 650 Hz. The phonocardiograms were recorded using a phonopre-amplifier (EMI 22) with electrical filters that together with a piezoelectric microphone (EMI 25 C) gave six frequency ranges including one aural frequency range. The pulse tracings and apex cardiograms were obtained using crystal transducers (EMI 510 C) with low frequency time constants between 1.9 and 4.6 s (depending on a capacitance-resistance product, decided by the individual amplification used for each curve) and connected by a 25 to 40 cm rubber tube to a specially designed capillary-damped funnel pick-up, 2.5 cm in diameter, giving a frequency response of at least 0.08 (at low frequency time constant 1.9 s) to 65 Hz (-3dB) (29). The paper speed was 50 mm/s for the electrocardiogram and for the other tracings 100 mm/s.

Simultaneous recordings of electrocardiogram lead II, a
phono-cardiogram from the third left intercostal space para-
sternally, a carotid pulse tracing or apex cardiogram were
recorded during the resting period proceding the measurement of
resting blood pressure. The carotid pulse tracing was recorded
in the supine position and the apex cardiogram in the left lateral
positon, both during relaxed expiratory apnea.

All channels were corrected for coincidence, the deviations
being calculated as the mean value of the difference in upstroke
in 4 consecutive mV tests induced simulataneously in the 7
channels. Correction was also made for the time delay (4 ms)
in the recording system (29). The measurement points were
determined in relation to 4 arbitrary reference lines (Fig. 1)

The time intervals studied (Fig. 1, lower panel) were as
follows:-

1. Total electromechanical systole from the beginning of the
    QRS complex to the beginning of the aortic component of the
    second heart sound (QA_2).

2. The electromechanical interval from the beginning of the
    QRS complex to the systolic upstroke of the apex cardiogram
    (EMI). In 4 subjects (11%) in the reference group, 1
    hypertensive subject (5%), and 1 patient in the infarct group
    (1.5%) an acceptable apex cardiogram could not be recorded,
    and in another 2 subjects in the reference group and 1 in
    the infarct group the upstroke of the apex cardiogram could
    not be identified with certainty.

3. The left ventricular ejection time from the beginning of the
    systolic upstroke of the carotid pulse tracing to the
    incisura (LVET). The LVET was also expressed as a percentage
    of the expected value for the given heart rate calculated
    from the regression equation between LVET and heart rate in
    the reference group (LVET%).

4. The pre-ejection period (PEP = QA_2-LVET).

5. The isovolumetric contraction time (ICT = PEP-EMI).

6. The PEP/LVET ratio).

7. The ICT/LVET ratio.

8. The interval between A_2 and the point on the downstroke of
    the apex cardiogram at which the curve fell to 10 per cent
    of the total height of the curve (A_2-90% amplitude reduction.

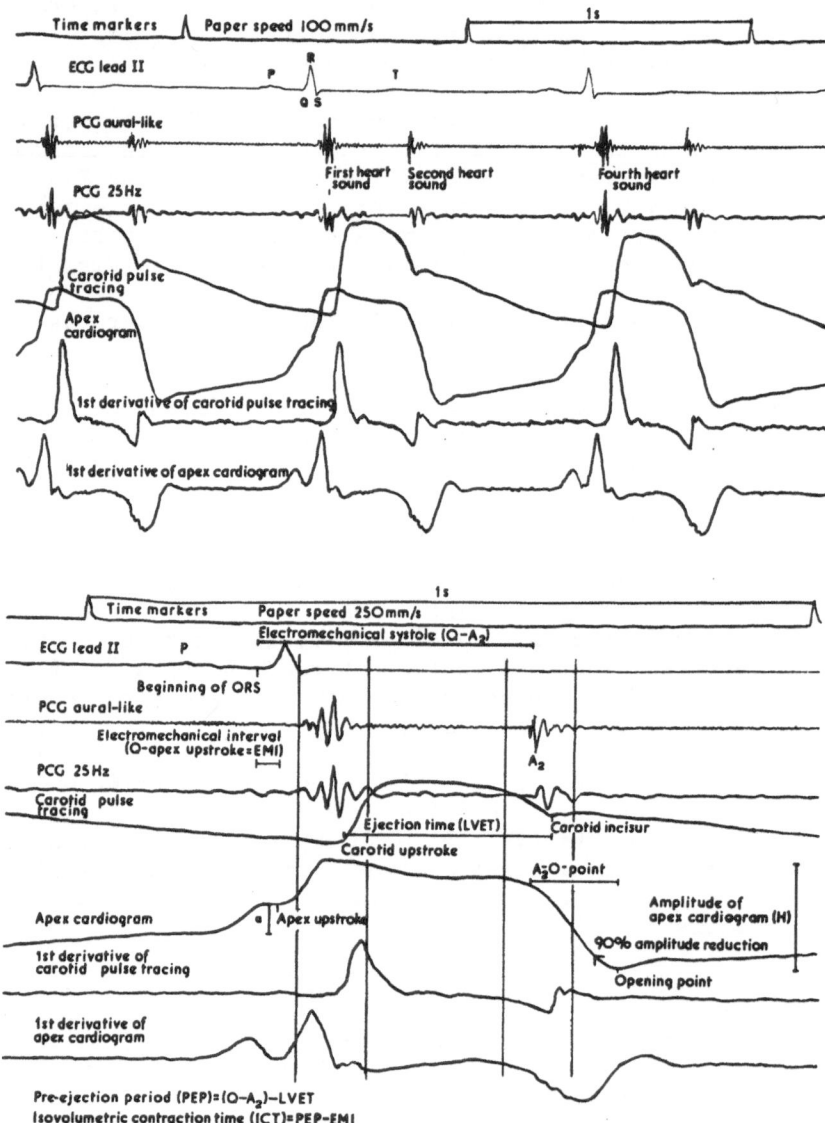

Figure 1.

Fig. 1.   Simultaneous recording of the apex cardiogram, carotid
          pulse tracing, phonocardiogram, and electrocardiogram in
          one of the infarct patients. Upper panel: paper speed
          100 mm/s. Lower panel: time intervals are, for practical
          reasons, marked on this recording at a paper speed of
          250 mm/s. Four reference lines (marked in lower panel,
          were used when the time intervals were measured (see
          Methods). The a-wave (a) and the total height (H) of
          the apex cardiogram are also marked in the lower panel
          (abbreviations, see Methods).

9.   The interval between the aortic component of the second
     sound and the O-point of the apex cardiogram (A_2O). In 3
     subjects in the reference group the O-point could not be
     identified with certainty.

     Limits for abnormal time intervals were arbitrarily set at
the second highest or lowest value in the reference group
depending on whether a high or low value of the variable concerned
was of pathological significance. If the two highest (or lowest)
values in the reference group were identical, the limit was set
at the highest (or lowest) value. On this vasis pathological
values were defined as: EMI⩾40ms, PEP⩾130 ms, ICT⩾100 mm,
LVET⩽90 per cent, ICT/LVET>0.35, PEP/LVET>0.45, A_2 to 90 per cent
amplitude reduction⩾105 ms, and A_2O⩾150 ms. The diastolic resting
blood pressure was divided by the ICT and in a corresponding
manner a diastolic blood pressure/ICT⩽775 mmHg/s was defined as
pathologically low. The limit for elevation of this variable
was set at 1200 mmHg/s.

RESULTS

     EMI was longer (P<0.01) in the infarct group ($\bar{x}$ = 34 ms) than
in the reference group ($\bar{x}$ = 27 ms), Table 1.

     There were no significant differences in means between the groups
with respect to ICT or PEP (Table 1).

     There was no difference in the mean value for LVET between
the three groups.

     Combination of systolic time intervals. Altogether 10 per
cent of the patients in the infarct group and 11 per cent of the
hypertensives had values of ICT⩾100 ms or LVET⩽90 per cent which
are not significantly higher than in the reference group, 3 per
cent (Table 2). The discrimination was not improved in the
variable ICT/LVET was added and no patient with normal values for
ICT, LVET, or ICT/LVET had an abnormal PEP/LVET value. There
were no significant differences in means between the groups with
respect of ICT/LVET or PEP/LVET.

TABLE 1.

Summary of means (ms) of time interval measurements

Measurement	Reference group n=36	Hypertensive group n=18	Infarct group n=67
$Q - A_2$	397	397	410
EMI	27	31	34
PEP	104	104	107
ICT	77	74	73
LVET	293	293	300
$A_2 - 0$	133	153	160
Rest. SBP	123	154	124
Rest. DBP	77	96	81
Heart rate	60	61	61

TABLE 2.

Proportion of subjects with isovolumetric contraction time ICT$\geqslant$ 100 ms, left ventricular ejection time LVET$\leqslant$90 per cent, and ICT/LVET>0.35 in the 3 groups

	Reference group		Hypertensive group		Infarct group	
	n	%	n	%	n	%
ICT $\geqslant$ 100 ms	1/30	3	1/18	6	4/63	6
LVET $\leqslant$ 90%	0/36	0	1/19	5	4/67	6
ICT/LVET > 0.35	1/30	3	1/18	6	2/63	3
Cumulative total	1/36	3	2/19	11	7/67	10

Only 4 infarct patients (6%) had pressure rise velocities (= diastolic blood pressure divided by ICT) below 775 mmHg/s.

The mean pressure rise velocity was higher (p<0.01) in the hypertensive group ($\bar{x}$ = 1323 mmHg/s) than in the reference group ($\bar{x}$ = 1044 mmHg/s). In the infarct group the mean value was 1168 mmHg/s. Sixty-seven per cent of the men in the hypertensive group and 38 per cent of the infarct patients had pressure rise velocities >1200 mmHg/s, which was more (p<0.01) than in the reference group (4%). When infarct patients who were taking digitalis or beta-blockers were excluded from this analysis 34 patients remained. Thirty-two per cent of these patients showed values of pressure rise velocity above 1200 mmHg/s, which was still more (p<0.02) than in the reference group.

The A_2O interval was longer (p<0.01) in both the hypertensive group ($\bar{x}$ = 153 ms) and the infarct group ($\bar{x}$ = 160 ms) than in the reference group ($\bar{x}$ = 133 ms). The proportion of patients with A_2O interval 150 ms was also higher (p<0.01) in the hypertensive group (56%) and the infarct group (74%) than in the reference group, 3 per cent.

DISCUSSION

When cardiac function has been studied more precisely in hypertensives or infarct patients this has previously been done in small selected groups of hospital patients, the control groups also necessarily being small and selected. To avoid the drawbacks entailed by selection the groups in the present study comprised random population samples. The results showed that only the electromechanical interval, pressure rise velocity, and A_2O point interval were useful discriminants between the three groups. It is clear that invasive assessment of left ventricular function would have yielded interesting data for correlation with the non-invasive data. Catheterisation and angiocardiography were, however, not performed, as it was not considered ethically justifiable to perform these invasive investigations in the symptomless subjects in the reference and hypertensive groups derived by screening, or in several of the infarct patients. Several studies of the correlation between non-invasive variables and invasive indices of left ventricular function have been carried out by other authors in selected groups of subjects (23, 15, 22).

Comparison of the mean values for systolic time intervals. in the infarct and hypertensive groups with those in the reference group showed that the pattern was not that which could be expected when left ventricular function was impaired. The prognostic value was difficult to assess since the number of infarct patients who died during follow-up was low and very

few infarct patients had divergent systolic time intervals. The
prognostic value of the combined non-invasive data is discussed
elsewhere, the systolic time intervals having been found in several
cases to be quite normal despite the fact that other non-invasive
data suggested considerable impairment of left ventricular function
(28). Furthermore, 3 of the 4 infarct patients with low LVET
were taking digitalis. Digitalis shortens LVET even in patients
with heart failure (26), and the significance of a shortened
LVET is thus difficult to assess in a patient taking digitalis.

A quarter of the patients in the infarct group had prolonged
EMI values, indicating delayed start of the systolic contraction
of the left ventricle (33, 14). An individual with apparently
normal impulse conduction on the electrocardiogram may thus
have a prolonged PEP, owing to prolongation of the EMI, which may
be erroneously interpreted as indicating a prolonged isovolumetric
contraction time. Even complicated and sophisticated invasive
isovolumetric indices of left ventricular function have proved
to be of doubtful value (17, 12).

It has been found that the diagnostic value of the PEP
increases when it is combined with invasively measured pulmonary
capillary venous pressure and non-invasively measured diastolic
arterial blood pressure for calculation of the pressure rise
velocity in the left ventricle (1, 6). Combination of ICT and
resting diastolic arterial blood pressure did not improve
discrimination in our study as regards impaired left ventricular
function.

Infarct patients exhibit signs of increased sympathetic
activity in the acute phase, which can be reduced by beta-blockade
(24). Our data regarding pressure rise velocity suggest that the
sympathetic activity may be raised in these patients at rest even
long after the acute phase. The results showed that the pressure
rise velocity during the isovolumetric contraction was also
higher in hypertensives than in normotensive individuals. This
was at least partly related to left ventricular hypertrophy as
judged by orthogonal electrocardiogram (28).

It has been claimed that arterial pressure must be included
as a prime determinant of LVET along with stroke volume, heart
rate, and inotropic state in man (20). Our results accord,
however, with the findings of Weissler et al (25), that among
patients with chronic arterial hypertension and minimal functional
impairment no independent effect of arterial pressure on the
systolic time intervals or PEP/LVET ration can be shown. Braunwald
et al (5) have also shown that when heart rate and stroke volume
were maintained constant, increasing aortic pressure did not
affect the duration of ejection except at very high mean aortic
pressure (175 to 200 mmHg).

The results regarding the systolic time intervals give the impression that the hypertensive group as well as the infarct group were homogeneous. It is, however, obvious from other non-invasive results in these groups that the nature as well as the severity of heart involvement varies considerably within the groups (4, 27-28) though the systolic time intervals failed to show this. Signs of systolic left ventricular functional impairment appear at a late stage since the altered filling pattern during diastole, with powerful atrial contractions and increased diastolic filling and hypertrophy of the left ventricle, may for a long time compensate for the impaired left ventricular function, at least during rest (19,7). When impairment of the left ventricular function is studied at an early stage interest should, therefore, be concentrated mainly on diastole. Several methods are required to identify the majority of patients with left ventricular dysfunction and the systolic time intervals are only a small part of the whole picture.

The A_2O interval was significantly prolonged in more than 50 per cent of the hypertensives and more than 70 per cent of the patients in the infarct group. The finding that not only the A_2O interval but also the interval between A_2 and a point on the diastolic downstroke of the apex cardiogram defined by the total amplitude of the apex cardiogram discriminates well between the groups, supports the postulate that this phase of the cardiac cycle really was prolonged. One of the reasons why such a striking finding has been so little studied may be the use of transducers with too short low frequency time constants in many previous studies, since transducers with short low frequency time constants not only shorten the A_2O interval but also tend to smooth out differences between an individual with a prolonged, and a person with a normal, A_2O interval (29).

Previously the A_2O interval has often been used as a synonym for the isovolumetric relaxation time (3, 9). The A_2O interval, however, comprises two phases, the relaxation phase and a period of the early filling phase of the left ventricle. Since the mean value for this filling phase has been calculated to be 50 ms (18), the latter may in certain cases represent about one-third of the A_2O interval. Further studies are required to elucidate the reasons for the prolongation of the A_2O interval in hypertensives and in postinfarction patients.

References

1. C. M. Agress, S. Wegner, J. S. Forrester, K. Chatterjee, W. W. Parmley, and H. J. C. Swan. An indirect method for evaluation of left ventricular function in acute myocardial infarction. Circulation 46:291-297 (1972).

2. S. S. Ahmed, G. E. Levinson, C. J. Schwartz, and P. O. Ettinger: Systolic time intervals as measures of the contractile state of the left ventricular myocardium.in man. Circulation 46: 559-571 (1972).

3. A. Benchimol, and J. G. Ellis: A study of the period of isovolumetric relaxation in normal subjects and in patients with heart disease. American Journal of Cardiology 19: 196-206 (1967).

4. G. Berglund, J. Wikstrand, I. Wallentin, and L. Wilhelmsen: Sodium excretion and sympathetic activity in relation to severity of hypertensive disease. Lancet 1: 324-328 (1976).

5. E. Braunwald, S. J. Sarnoff, and W. N. Stainsby: Determinants of duration and mean rate of ventricular ejection. Circulation Research 6: 319-325 (1958).

6. G. Diamond, J. S. Forrester, K. Chatterjee, S. Wegner, and H. J. C. Swan: Mean electromechanical $\Delta P/\Delta t$. An indirect index of the peak rate of rise of left ventricular pressure. American Journal of Cardiology 30: 338-342 (1972).

7. H. T. Dodge: Haemodynamic aspects of cardiac failure. In The Myocardium: Failure and Infarction, p.70 E. Braunwald, ed., HP Publishing Co., New York, (1973).

8. C. L. Garrard, A. M. Weissler, and H. T. Dodge: The relationship of alterations in systolic time intervals to ejection fraction in patients with cardiac disease. Circulation 42: 455-462 (1970).

9. D. Harmjanz, D. Böttcher, and G. Schertlein: Correlations of electrocardiographic pattern, shape of ventricular septum, and isovolumetric relaxation time in irregular hypertrophic cardiomyopathy (obstructive cardiomyopathy). British Heart Journal 33: 928-937 (1971).

10. M. Hodges, B. L. Halpern, G. C. Friesinger, and G. R. Degenais: Left ventricular pre-ejection period and ejection time in patients with acute myocardial infarction. Circulation 45: 933-942 (1972).

11. J. M. Johnson, W. Siegel, and G. Blomqvist: Characteristics of transducers used for recording the apexcardiogram. Journal of Applied Physiology, 31: 796-800 (1971).

12. T. H. Kreulen, A. A. Bove, M. T. McDonough, M. J. Sands, and J. F. Spann: The evaluation of left ventricular function in man,. A comparison of methods. Circulation 51: 677-688 (1975).

13. S. Kumar, and D. H. Spodick: Study of the mechanical events of the left ventricle by atraumatic techniques: comparison of methods of measurement and their significance. American Heart Journal, 80: 401-413 (1970).

14. J. Manolas, W. Rutishauser, P. Wirz, and U. Arbenz: Time relation between apex cardiogram and left ventricular events using simultaneous high-fidelity tracings in man. British Heart Journal, 37: 1263-1267 (1975)

15. C. E. Martin, J. A. Shaver, M. E. Thompson, P. S. Reddy, and J. J. Leonard: Direct correlation of external systolic time

intervals with internal indices of left ventricular function
in man. Circulation, 44: 419-431 (1971).

16. M. E. Parker, and H. G. Just: Systolic time intervals in
    coronary artery disease as indices of left ventricular
    function: fact or fancy? British Heart Journal, 36:
    368-376 (1974).

17. K. L. Peterson, D. Skloven, P. Ludbrook, J. B. Uther, and
    J. Ross: Comparison of isovolumetric and ejection phase
    indices of myocardial performance in man. Circulation, 49:
    1088-1101 (1974).

18. T. Prewitt, D. Gibson, D. Brown, and G. Sutton: The 'rapid
    filling wave' of the apex cardiogram. British Heart Journal
    37: 1256-1262 (1975).

19. C. E. Rackley, W. P. Hood, E. L. Rolett, and D. T. Young:
    Left ventricular end-diastolic pressure in chronic heart
    disease. American Journal of Medicine, 48:310-319 (1970).

20. J. A. Shaver, F. W. Kroetz, J.J. Leonard, and H. W. Paley:
    The effect of steady-state increases in systemic arterial
    pressure on the duration of left ventricular ejection time.
    Journal of Clinical Investigation, 47: 217-230 (1968).

21. M. E. Tavel, R. W. Campbell, H. Feigenbaum, and E. F.
    Steinmetz: The apex cardiogram and its relationship to
    haemodynamic events within the left heart. British Heart
    Journal, 27: 829-839 (1965).

22. F. van de Werf, J. Piessens, H. Kesteloot, and H. de Geest:
    A comparison of systolic time intervals derived from the
    central aortic pressure and from the external carotid pulse
    tracing. Circulation, 51: 310-316 (1975).

23. G. C. Voigt, and G. C. Friesinger: The use of apex cardio-
    graphy in the assessment of left ventricular diastolic
    pressure. Circulation, 41: 1015-1024 (1970).

24. F. Waagstein, A. C. Hjalmarson, and H. S. Wasir: Apex
    cardiogram and systolic time intervals in acute myocardial
    infarction and effects of practolol. British Heart Journal
    36: 1109-1121 (1974).

25. A. M. Weissler, W. S. Harris, and C. D. Schoenfeld: Bedside
    technics for the evaluation of ventricular function in man.
    American Journal of Cardiology 23: 577-583 (1969).

26. A. M. Weissler, and C. D. Schoenfeld: Effect of digitalis on
    systolic time intervals in heart failure. American Journal
    of the Medical Sciences, 259: 4-20 (1970).

27. J. Wikstrand: Non-invasive assessment of cardiac function.
    Studies in normotensive and hypertensive 50-year-old men
    and male infarction patients aged 48-57. Thesis Göteborg,
    Sweden. (Available on request).

28. J. Wikstrand, G. Berglund, L. Wilhelmsen, and I. Wallentin:
    Orthogonal electrocardiogram, apex cardiogram, and atrial
    sound in normotensive and hypertensive 50-year-old men.
    British Heart Journal, 38: 779-789 (1976).

29. J. Wikstrand, K. Nilsson, and I. Wallentin: Distortion of
    non-invasive cardiac pulse curves. A capillary-damped pick-up
    and a calibration unit for apex cardiograms and other pulse
    curves. British Heart Journal, 39: 995-1005 (1977).
30. J. Wikstrand, G. Berglund, L. Wilhelmsen, and I. Wallentin:
    Value of systolic and diastolic time intervals. Studies in
    normotensive and hypertensive 50-year-old men and in patients
    after myocardial infarction. British Heart Journal, 40:
    256-267 (1978).
31. L. Wilhelmsen, G. Berglund, and L. Werkö: Prevalence and
    management of hypertension in a general population sample of
    Swedish men. Preventive Medicine, 2: 57-66 (1973).
32. L. Wilhelmsen, G. Tibblin, and L. Werkö: A primary preventive
    study in Gothenburg, Sweden. Preventive Medicine, 1: 153-160
    (1972).
33. J. L. Willems, H. de Geest, and H. Kesteloot: On the value of
    apex cardiography for timing intracardiac events. American
    Journal of Cardiology, 28: 59-66 (1971).

PLATELET AGGREGATION, COAGULATION AND FIBRINOLYSIS AT REST

AND AFTER BICYCLE ERGOMETER TEST IN CHD

A. Strano, S. Novo, G. Davi', G. Avellone, and A. Pinto

Clinica Medica I
University of Palermo
Italy

Several observers have suggested that a dysfunction of dynamic balance between platelet aggregation, coagulation and fibrinolysis may be a factor in the pathogenesis of atherosclerosis. This dysfunction, presumably, is correlated with the atherosclerotic vascular lesions, that could reduce the parietal synthesis of heparan-sulphase, prostacyclin and plas minogen activator.

A thrombophilic state can, so, favour the development and the progression of degenerative atherosclerotic changes and the occlusion of the atherosclerotic artery. In fact, platelets might play a part in atherogenesis(26) and further might initiate arterial thrombosis or by aggregating at the side of previous vascular injury or activating the coagulation factors(30) that in presence of impaired fibrinolysis favour the deposition of fibrin.

Exercise induce coagulation balance changes; in healthy it performed a moderate activation of coagulative factors and platelet aggregation with an increase of plasmatic fibrinolytic activity (3-4-6-14-29). Therefore, the magnitude of fibrinolytic response to exercise is reduced in patients with atherosclerosis and diurnal fibrinolytic response is impaired in patients with CHD (19-23-24).

It appears that the mechanism of stress or exercise-induced coagulative changes is via the release of endogenous cathecolamines and numerous epidemiological studies have demonstrated that coronary atherosclerosis and acute myocardial infarction occur in men that are subject to acute and recurrent stress(20-25). Infusion of sympathetic catecholamines, also, will increase the

stickness of platelets and will cause platelet aggregation in
myocardial small vessels(11-12-13).

Haerem(8-9-10) reported that platelet aggregates in the
epicardial coronary arteries of patients who died suddenly or
cardiac causes were more numerous and larger than those found in
patients without cardial disease.

Levites and Haft(16) determined that exercise increases
significantly the tendency of platelets to aggregate among patients
with coronary artery disease; this increased platelet aggregability
is restored toward normal with propranolol in dosage sufficient to
improve exercise tolerance(7).

The alteration of haemostasis during exercise, more evident in
patients with CHD, induce to investigate the coagulative homeostasis
in those patients that must improve cardiac performance with a
rehabilitation program. The coagulative changes pay play a role in
angina pectoris or myocardial infarction induced during physical
work. Platelets, during aggregation, release thromboxa e A_2, which
is potent in costricting coronary smooth muscle with S-T segment
changes, in laboratory animals(18); recently Maseri(17) documented
that, in some cases, a persistent coronary spasm can induce
myocardial infarction.

However, an increased platelet aggregability with a coagulative
activation and a reduced fibrinolytic response might cause intravascular thrombi further narrowing the lumen of sclerotic
coronary vessels.

Our research, carried out on patients with ischemic heart
disease and healthy subjects, matched for sex and age, was undertaken to define if a standard exercise test will affect, in
different manner, the propensity for platelet to aggregate, the
modifications of the coagulative factors and the magnitudo of
fibrinolytic response in the two groups.

Materials and Methods

Ten hospitalized patients, with stable angina pectoris and
positive bicycle ergometer test and ten healthy subjects, age and
sex matched, were included in this study. They were 4 women and
6 men with age ranging from 45 to 60 years.

After a preliminary screening were excluded the patients with
diabetes, hypertension, cardiac failure, LBBB, RBBB, myocardial
infarction and severe arrhytmias (auricolar fibrillation,
auricolar flutter and ventricular premature beats).

All patients remained in bed from 10 p.m. to 8 a.m.; blood samples were drawn at 8 a.m. at bed rest, then in the ergometer laboratory were drawn at the end of exercise and 30' after the exercise.

Blood samples were obtained from an ante-decubital vein in such a manner that blood flowed freely from an 18-gauge needle into a killed glass centrifuge tube containing 3,2% trisodium citrate diydrate (one part citrate; nine parts blood); another blood sample was collected in a killed glass centrifuge tube without citrate. Samples were refrigerated and brought to the laboratory in an ice-cooled container.

Euglobulin lysis time was detected using the method of Von Kaulla modified(21-27). Alpha-1-antitrypsin and alpha-2-macroglobulin were performed by immunodiffusion radial plates using the Mancini e Carbonara method(2). The primary antiplasmin was determined by Collen method(5). The antithrombin III biological activity was detected in according to Von Kaulla method(28). A PTT was determined using Biochemia-Kit.Platelet aggregation studies were performed using the turbidometric method of Born(1) on PR adjusted to the range 300.000-400.000 mm^3, evaluating the maximal rate of aggregation and the threshold of irreversible aggregation to ADP, the collagen-lag period. The platelet count ratio, according to Wu and Hoak(31) was also used.

Bicycle ergometer test was performed, utilizing the Redwood protocol(22), until chest pain for the patients and at the same work load for matched subjects. The electrocardiogram was monitoring continuously with an oscilloscope and blood pressure and electrocardiographic rhythm strips were obtained at one minute into each stage of the protocol, at the conclusion and 5', 10', 15' into the recovery period.

RESULTS

In the control subjects (CS), at rest, the mean euglobulin lysis time (ELT) was 181,72 $\pm$ 106,5 minutes, significantly lower than did patients with angina pectoris (AP), 410,5 $\pm$ 90,37 min. (p.< 0.0005) (Fig. 1).

At the conclusion of exercise, ELT decreased to 100,1 $\pm$ 76,74 min. in CS and to 300,08 $\pm$ 67,43 min. in AP (p<0.0005); 30' after exercise ELT was 88,5 $\pm$ 56,2 in CS and 271,66 $\pm$ 69,09 min. in AP (p<0.0005). The percentage change between ELT at rest and at conclusion of exercise (fig.2) was 44,9 $\pm$ 10,6% in CS and 26,9 $\pm$ 6,4% in AP; 30' after exercise the mean variation of the ELT activity was 51,5 $\pm$ 11,7% in CS and 33,84 $\pm$ 7,3% in AP.

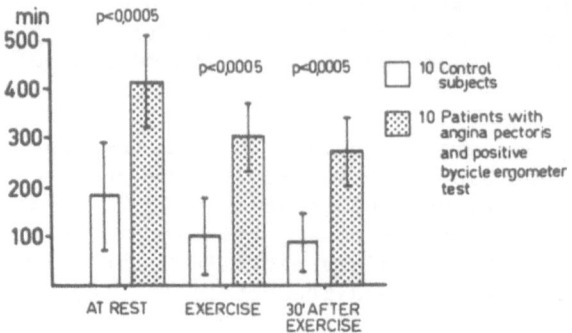

Fig. 1.   Euglobulin lysis time

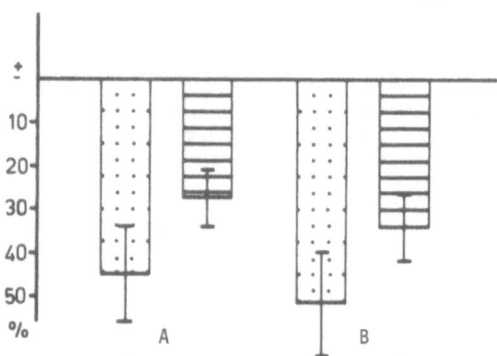

Fig. 2.   Percentage changes in E.L.T. (A) between exercise and
rest and (B) between 30 minutes after exercise and rest
in control subjects [··] and in patients with angina
pectoritis and positive bicycle ergometer test [≡]

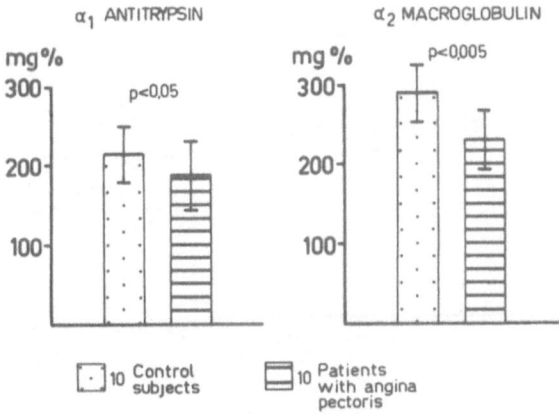

Figure 3.

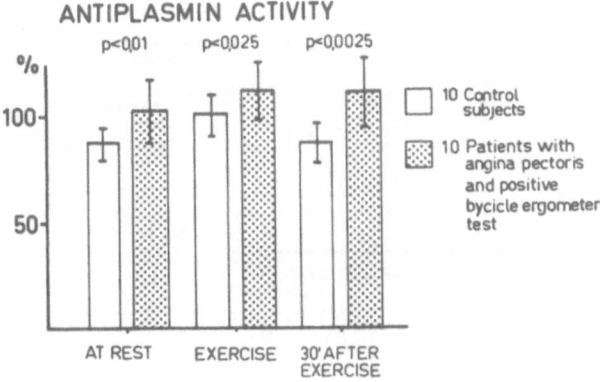

Figure 4.

Alpha-1-antitrypsin, at rest, was 216,4 $\pm$ 33,2 mg % in CS (fig. 3) and 188,5 $\pm$ 42,3 mg % in AP (p<0.05); also alpha-2-macroglobulin levels was greater in CS (291,6 $\pm$ 34,8 mg %) than in AP (230,4 $\pm$ 37,6 mg %) (p<0.0005).

Figure 4 shows that CS had a significantly lower mean anti-plasmin activity (88,00 $\pm$ 7,9 %), at rest, than did AP (103,49 $\pm$ 14,45%; p<0.01). The increase of antiplasmin activity in AP was also evident at conclusion of exercise (101 $\pm$ 9,1 %) that in CS (113,33 $\pm$ 13,8 %) (p<0.025) and 30' after exercise (88 $\pm$ 8,3 % in CS and 112,2 $\pm$ 16,28 % in AP - p<0.0025).

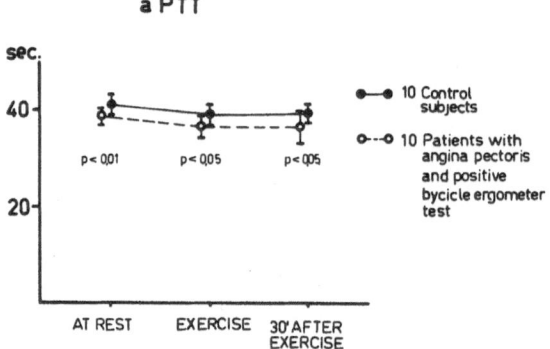

Figure 5.

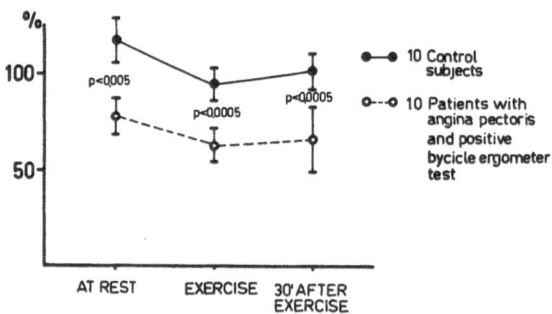

Figure 6.

   The aPTT (fig. 5), at rest, showed lower levels in AP
(38,56 ± 1,72 sec.) that in CS (41,03 ± 2,15 sec. - p<0.01) and
the same change was observed at conclusion of exercise (36,76 ±
1,48 sec in AP and 39,01 ± 2,01 sec in CS - p<0.05) and 30' after
exercise (36,57 ± 3,35 sec in AP and 39,08 ± 1,9 sec in CS -
p<0.05).

   Figure 6 shows that the patients with angina pectoris had a
significantly lower mean biological activity of antithrombin III
(67,12 ± 9,28 %), at rest, than did CS (117,12 ± 10,2 % - p<0.005);
after exercise the AP did not show the same consistent decreases
in antithrombin III activity (62,2 ± 8,75 %) that were observed in
CS (94,98 ± 8,7 % - p<0.0005) also the same change were achieved
30' after exercise (65,92 ± 17,18 in AP and 101,15 ± 9,3 in CS
- p<0.0005).

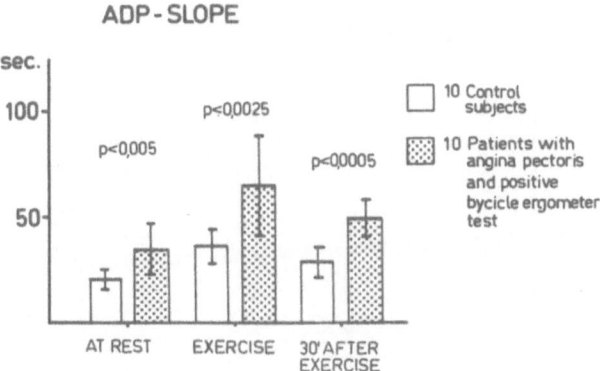

Figure 7.

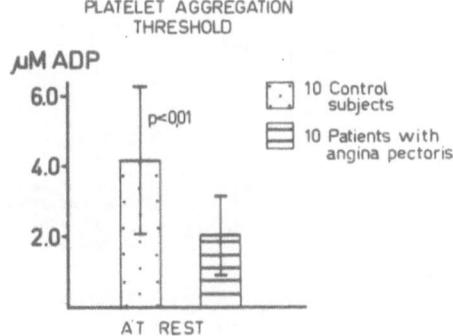

Figure 8.

The slope (fig. 7), using 1,25 micromoli ADP, was, at rest, 20,08 $\pm$ 4,1 sec for CS and 34,0 $\pm$ 11,53 sec for AP (p<0.005). At peak work this value increased to 36,25 $\pm$ 7,8 sec for CS and to 65,33 $\pm$ 23,18 sec for AP (p<0.0005); 30' after exercise the slope was 49,33 $\pm$ 8,32 sec for CS and 29,18 $\pm$ 6,4 sec for AP (p<0.0005). The mean concentration required to produce the threshold aggregation response was 4,16 $\pm$ 2,09 micromoli ADP for CS and 2,01 $\pm$ 1,10 micromoli ADP for AP (p<0.01) (fig. 8).

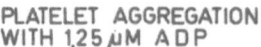
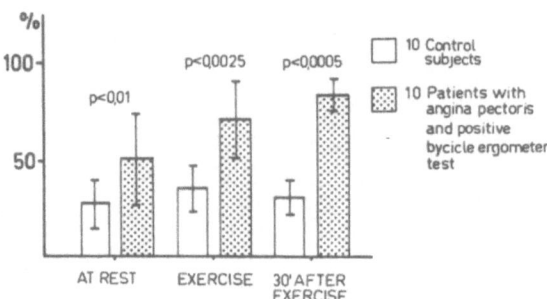

Figure 9.

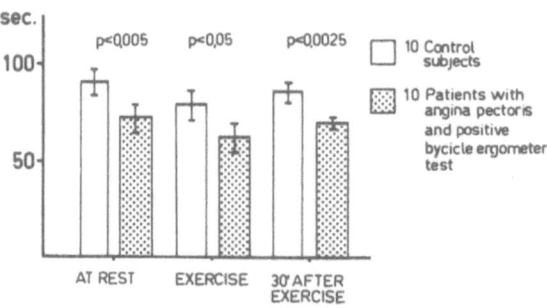

Figure 10.

The changes in percent of aggregation using 1,25 microM ADP, was 28,8 $^+_-$ 10,2% for the control group and 51,49 $^+_-$ 23 % for the patients with AP, at rest, (p 0.01) at conclusion of exercise 35,9 $^+_-$ 11,6 % for CS and 71,09 $^\pm$ 19,66 % for AP (p 0.0025), 30' after exercise it was 84, 78 $^\pm$ 7,58 % for AP (p 0.0005) and 30,22 $\pm$ 8,4 % for CS (fig. 9).

The collagen-lag period (at the concentration of 200 ng) was at rest, 91,34 $^\pm$ 51 sec in CS and 72,9 $^\pm$ 7,1 sec in AP (p 0.005), at conclusion of the exercise 79,32 $^+_-$ 7,1 sec in CS and 62,5 $^+_-$ 6,92 sec in AP (p 0.05), 30' after exercise 86,5 $^+_-$ 4,4 sec in CS and 69,6 $\pm$ 2,64 sec in AP (p 0.0025). (fig. 10).

The mean platelet count ratio, at rest, was 0,96 $\pm$ 0.02 for CS and 0,91 $\pm$ 0.02 for the stable angina group (p<0.0005), at conclusion of exercise 0.81 $\pm$ 0,07 for CS and 0,75 $\pm$ 0.05 (p<0.01) for AP, 30' after exercise 0,92 $\pm$ 0.03 for CS and 0,80 $\pm$ 0.03 for AP (p<0.0005). (Fig. 11).

Discussion

In the present study we have demonstrated, yet at rest, a thrombophilic syndrome in patients with stable angina.

In fact, we have found a coagulative activation (reduced levels of At III), and an enhancement in platelet aggregability (increased platelet circulating aggregates; more irreversible aggregation responses to ADP and collagen) and a depression of fibrinolytic system with a longer euglobulin lysis time and an increased activity of primary antiplasmin.

The platelet aggregagability and the coagulative processes were significantly enhanced immediately following the exercise test, balanced in the controls,by an activation of fibrinolysis. In the patients with stable angina, after exercise, is more evident the coagulative activation and the platelet hyperaggregability with a reduced response of the fibrinolytic activity. The changes of the coagulative homeostasis in the patients with stable angina may be a catecholamine-mediated effect together with a reduced production of antithrombotic substances by the atherosclerotic vessel wall.

Therefore, the precipitating event in myocardial infarction or in stable angina, during a period of stress or exercise, could be a catecholamine-mediated phenomenon, inducing intra-arterial platelet aggregates capable of occluding already narrowed segments of the coronary circulation (15).

Our data suggest that in patients with stable angina that must undergo towards a rehabilitation program, it's useful the study of the coagulative system to demonstrate the possible thrombophilic syndrome and so associate a therapy with antithrombotic drugs.

SUMMARY

In atherosclerotic patients is frequently found an augmented coagulation and platelet activity with a reduced fibrinolysis. These altered haemostatic balance could favour the thrombotic evolution of this atherosclerotic lesions; but some AA. think that an enhanced platelet aggregation can play a role also in initial atherosclerotic lesions.

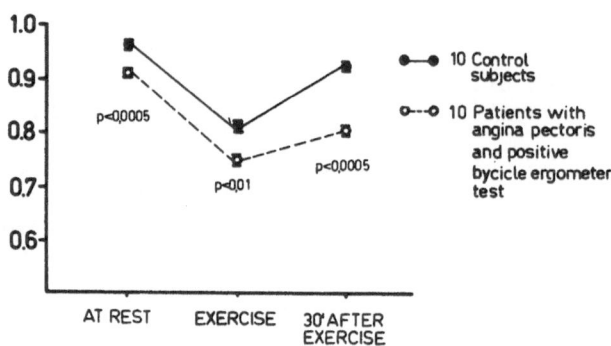

Figure 11.

The exercise, in the normal, induces release of catecholamines these substances augment contractile activity and O_2 consumption of myocardium and also induce an exalted coagulation and platelet activity but increase fibrinolytic activity.

Therefore, it's very interesting to know if it is possible to observe these modifications in patients with coronary heart disease. Of course, an exalted platelet activity induced by exercise could, in a patient with angina pectoris, favour coronary spasm by production of thromboxane A_2, released during the platelet aggregation. There are not many works about this argument, but it is possible to think that in patients with coronary heart disease, during exercise, is more evident the exalted platelet and coagulation activity with hypofibrinolysis.

Also our researches, in patients with CHD, evaluating some parameters (platelet aggregation induced by ADP and collagen, At III,. euglobulin lysis time, antiplasmin plasmatic activity, at rest, and after exercise with bicycle ergometer till angor induction, seem to demonstrate a marked platelet and coagulation activity with a poor response of the fibrinolytic system.

The alterations of the coagulation system could favour the evolution of myocardial ischemia.

References

1. G. V. R. Born, Quantitative investigation into the aggregation of platelets, J. Physiol, 20:423 (1965)
2. O. Carbonara, G. Mancini, Techniche di immunodiffusione per il dosaggio delle proteine, La Ricerca in Clin. e Lab. suppl. 1:151 (1970).
3. J. D. Cash, Effects of moderate exercise on the fibrinolytic system in normal young men and women, Br. Med. J. 2:502 (1966).
4. F. D'Onofrio, L. Coppola, A. Tirelli, R. Russo, L. Misso, M. Varricchio, Comportamento dell' aggregabilità piastrinica in soggetti normali e atero-arteriosclerotici dopo prova da sforzo al cicleorgometro, Atti Dell' European Symposium on Coagulation, Fibrinolysis, Platelet aggregation and Atherosclerosis, p.395, ed. Ceop, Roma (1978).
5. J. Edy, F. de Coock, D. Collen, Inhibition of plasmin by normal and antiplasmin depleted plasma, Throm. Res. 8:513 (1976).
6. A. Finkel, G. R. Cumming, Effects of exercise in the cold on blood clotting and platelets, J. Appl. Physiol, 5:549 (1970).
7. W. H. Frishman, B. Weksler, J. P. Christodoulou, C. Smithen, T. Killip, Reversal of a normal platelet aggregability and change in exercise tolerance in patients with angina pectoris following oral propanolol, Circ. 48:164 (1973).
8. J. W. Haerem, Sudden coronary death, the occurence of platelet aggregates in the epicardial arteries,Atherosclerosis 14:417 (1971).
9. J. W. Haerem, Platelet aggregates in intramyocardial vessels of patients dying suddenly and unexpectedly of coronary artery disease, Atherosclerosis 15:199 (1972).
10. J. W. Haerem. A role of platelet in the mechanism of myocardial infarction and sudden death, 7th European Congress of Cardiology Amsterdam (1976).
11. J. I. Haft, P. Kranz, F. Albert, K. Fani, Intravascular platelet aggregation in the heart induced by noreepinephrine; microscopic studies, Circ. 46:698 (1972).
12. J. I. Haft, K. Fani, Intravascular platelet aggregation in the heart induced by stress, Circ. 47:353 (1973).
13. J. I. Haft, K. Fani, Stress and the induction of intravascular platelet aggregation in the heart, Circ. 48:164 (1973).
14. S. G. Iatridis, J. H. Ferguson, Effect of physical exercise on blood clotting and fibrinolysis, J. Appl. Physiol. 18:353 (1973).
15. L. Jorgensen, H. C. Roswell, T. Hovig, M. F. Glynn, J. F. Mustard, Adenosine-diphosphate-induced platelet aggregation and myocardial infarction in Swine, Lab. Invest. 17:616 (1967).
16. R. Levites, J. I. Haft, Effects of exercise-induced stress on platelet aggregation, Cardiology 60:304 (1975).
17. A. Maseri, Coronary vasospasm, coronary atherosclerosis and acute myocardial ischemia. A possible vicious cycle, Intern. Conf. on Ather.,Milan, November 9-12 (1977).

18. S. Moncada, J. R. Vane, Arachidonic acid metabolites and interaction between platelets and blood-vessel walls, New Engl. J. Med. 1:1142 (1979).

19. R. T. Moxley, F. Brackman, T. Astrup, Resting levels of fibrinolysis in blood in inactive and exercising men, J. Appl. Physiol. 5:549 (1970).

20. P. J. Nestle, Relationship between blood fibrinolytic activity, serum lipoproteins, and serum cholesterol in atherosclerotic arterial disease, Austr. Ann. Med. 9:234 (1960).

21. S. Novo, G. Avellone, F. d'Eredita, A. Pinto, Il tempo di lisi delle euglobuline. Nota I: Comportamento in un gruppo di soggetti giovani sani in relazione al peso corporeo relativo, Boll. Soc. It. Cardiol., XXI, 12:2145 (1976).

22. D. R. Redwood, D. R. Rosing, R. E. Goldstein, G. D. Beiser, S. E. Epstein, Importance of the design of an exercise protocol in the valuation of patients with angina pectoris, Circ. 43:618 (1971).

23. D. R. Rosing, P. Brakman, D. R. Redweed, R. E. Goldstein, G. D. Beiser, T. Astrup, S. E. Epstein, Blood fibrinolytic activity: diurnal variation and response to varying level of exercise, Circ. Res. 27:171 (1970).

24. D. R. Rosing, D. R. Redwood, P. Brakeman, Impairment of the diurnal fibrinolytic response in man - Effect of aging, type IV hyperliproteinemia, and coronary artery disease, Circ. Res. 32:752 (1973).

25. H. I. Russek, B. I. Zohman, Relative significance of heredity, diet and occupational stress in coronary heart disease of young adults: based on analysis of 100 patients between the ages of 25 and 40 years and a similar group of 100 normal subjects, Am. J. Med. Sci. 235:266 (1968).

26. A. Strano. S. Novo, Prospettive sull'impiego degli antiaggreganti piastrinici nella prevenzione dell'aterosclerosi, Giorn. It. di Cardiol. IX, I, I,(1979).

27. K. N. Von Kaulla, Continous automatic recording of fibrin formation and fibrinolysis: a valuable method for coagulation research, J. Lab. Clin. Med. 49:304 (1957).

28. E. Von Kaulla, K. N. Von Kaulla, Antithrombin III and disease AM. J. Clin. Path. 48:69 (1967).

29. H. Yamazaki, T. Sano, T. Odakura, K. Takeuchi, T. Shimamoto, Electrocardiographic and hematological changes by exercise test in coronary patients and pyridinolcarbamate pretreatment. A double blind crossover trial, Am. Heart. J. 5:640 (1970).

30. P. N. Walsh, Platelet coagulant activities and haemostasis: a hypothesis. Blood 43:597 (1974).

31. K. K. Wu, J. C. Hoak, A new method for the quantitative detection of platelet aggregates in patients with arterial insufficiency, Lancet 2:924 (1974).

INDEX

Angina Pectoris
  circulatory measurements in,64
  physical training in, 59, 62
  threshold heart rate, 69
Angina unstable
  exercise test in, 42,43,47
Antithrombin activity
  exercise in, 270
Aortic valve motion, 237
Arrhythmias
  exercise and, 171
  exercise induced,209,211,212
    diagnostic implications of,
      213
    mechanism of, 210
    prognostic significance of,
      215
  holter monitoring during, 197
  life threatening, 138
  sub-maximal ergometry during,
    197

Beta blockers, 56
  exercise testing and, 170
  long term intervention, 145
  oxygen demand and, 149
  oxygen pulse and, 129
Blood pressure
  physical exertion at, 113

Calcium blockers, 57
Cardiocirculatory effect,
  prolonged training and, 66
Circulatory measurements,
  angina pectoris in, 64

Coagulation
  ergometry after, 265
Coronary bypass grafting, 133
  indications for, 139
  psychological aspect, 85
  rehabilitation after, 100

Diastolic time intervals, 253
Digitalis therapy
  heart volume and, 128
  oxygen pulse and, 128
Drugs
  antianginal, 53

Echocardiography
  exercise during, 240,241
  functional evaluation and,233
Ectopic cardiac activity
  mechanism of, 210, 211
Emotional reaction
  myocardial infarction to, 79
Enzymes oxidative, 62
Exercise electrocardiography,163
  comparison to angiography ,177
  triple vessel disease in, 187
Exercise testing
  arrhythmia and, 171
  arrhythmias induced by,209,211
    212
  drugs and, 40,45
  echocardiography, 240,241
  holter monitoring comparison,
    198,199,200
  in asymptomatic patients,178
  interpretation of, 43